For Linda,

and my other friends in the library.

Best Wishes. Michael Livingston

LISTENING IN MEDICINE

The Whiplash Mystery
And Other Tales

Thank you for all your help over the years.

MICHAEL LIVINGSTON

TRAFFORD
PUBLISHING

Note for Librarians: a cataloguing record for this book that includes Dewey Decimal Classification and US Library of Congress numbers is available from the Library and Archives of Canada. The complete cataloguing record can be obtained from their online database at: www.collectionscanada.ca/amicus/index-e.html

ISBN 1-4120-7169-0

Printed in Victoria, BC, Canada

Printed on paper with minimum 30% recycled fibre.

Trafford's print shop runs on "green energy" from solar, wind and other environmentally-friendly power sources.

TRAFFORD
PUBLISHING

Offices in Canada, USA, Ireland and UK

This book was published *on-demand* in cooperation with Trafford Publishing. On-demand publishing is a unique process and service of making a book available for retail sale to the public taking advantage of on-demand manufacturing and Internet marketing. On-demand publishing includes promotions, retail sales, manufacturing, order fulfilment, accounting and collecting royalties on behalf of the author.

Book sales for North America and international:

Trafford Publishing, 6E–2333 Government St.,

Victoria, BC v8t 4p4 CANADA

phone 250 383 6864 (toll-free 1 888 232 4444)

fax 250 383 6804; email to orders@trafford.com

Book sales in Europe:

Trafford Publishing (uk) Ltd., Enterprise House, Wistaston Road Business Centre,

Wistaston Road, Crewe, Cheshire cw2 7rp UNITED KINGDOM

phone 01270 251 396 (local rate 0845 230 9601)

facsimile 01270 254 983; orders.uk@trafford.com

Order online at:

trafford.com/05-2064

10 9 8 7 6 5

Other books by Michael Livingston

Family Medicine: an Inside Look (1980)

Back Aid (1982)

Beyond Backache (1988)

Common Whiplash Injury: A Modern Epidemic (1999)

CONTENTS

Keywords. Listening. Narrative Medicine. Family Medicine. History of Medicine. "Whiplash Injury". Insurance companies. Students in Health Sciences. Students in Social Sciences. Teachers.

FOREWORD

Dr. Livingston is a traditional doctor. In these days, so-called medically unexplained symptoms occupy a large part of medical consultations, both in family practice as well as in the specialties. Here it is clear that more, and more sophisticated, and more expensive investigations are not only unhelpful, but are often counter productive, increasing the patient's concerns with each negative result. Dr. Livingston proposes listening to the patient, and with magnificent examples illustrates the results that can be achieved by eliciting what the patient's real concerns are. He shows that even in the formal setting of an independent medical examination – where the physician allocates more time to interview the patient and to review the background material – information that provides a patient-centered therapeutic approach may also come forward, quite apart from what the lawyer/insurance company think about it. I don't think this process and the interpretation is as easy as he modestly implies, but he does show that the rewards would justify the effort of a trial for all of us.

As a specialist I have to believe that our arrival has advanced the science and practice of medicine very considerably. However, I also realize that it has led to fragmentation of care and often loss of the doctor/patient relationship. This loss may make it more than usually difficult to understand the patient's problems, and especially medically unexplained symptoms from a biopsychosocial model. This becomes particularly important when we recognize that, for example, depression is the most significant prognostic factor in explaining a bad outcome after myocardial infarction. Paradigms do change, but Dr. Livingston has shown that perhaps because of vested interests the idea that the so-called whiplash-associated disorders are due to an injury dies hard despite dramatic evidence to the contrary. For him it is the story that is important, the patient's own story, or that of the illness.

Anthony Russell MD. FRCP (C).
Professor of Medicine, Emeritus
University of Alberta, Edmonton, Alberta, Canada.

INTRODUCTION

Generally, current medical teaching neglects the importance of listening to patients. Students suffer from such neglect and their patients suffer later. So the following account emphasizes tales told by people to their doctors and aims to interest anyone studying, providing or receiving health care.

I offer evidence suggesting that patients' tales or narratives are central to understanding medicine and health care. I invite readers to consider the evidence, whether they be students in the health or social sciences, practitioners, teachers, insurance adjusters, lawyers, judges, health planners or general readers. Some of the writing is essentially social criticism. The observations follow from some 40 years of medical practice in British Columbia, Canada's most western province.

If this piece of history passes unreported it is lost forever.

I ask readers' forbearance for changes in style from narrative to expository and for the common use of the male gender. Small changes are made to prevent identification and to preserve patients' privacy.

In the beginning was the tale.

Just as tales told at the family's hearth and around the camp fire recorded the history of the family and of the tribe, so tales told by the sick to their healers and recorded by them enabled diagnoses to be made and treatment offered.

For example, four thousand years ago, an Egyptian practitioner, in his sparse records, described treating a patient who consulted him for a sprained neck, a "sprain in a cervical vertebra." [1] The patient told a brief tale, namely that he experienced pain in his neck when turning to look at his shoulders and at his breast. Noting his tale, the practitioner suggested,

"Thou shouldst bind it with meat the first day. Now afterward thou shouldst treat [with] YMRW (and) honey every day until he recovers."

Today, no-one knows what YMRW was.

Interestingly, the practitioner advised a greasy support with meat for one day only. The meat would have quickly deteriorated in Egypt's heat and attracted flies, thus discouraging the overuse of a "neck collar" and encouraging early restoration of movement, a concept returned to quite recently.[2,3] The Greek physician, Hippocrates, born on the tiny island of Cos about 460 B.C. and generally acknowledged to be the father of medicine, practised at a time when the popular causes of illness were thought to be the position of the stars, angry gods or magic. Seeking to find the real reasons people became ill he focused upon the patient's tale. For example,[4] in Epidemics III , Case VII, he noted where the patient lived, her initial sore throat, later parched tongue, high fever, rigours and a reddish hard swelling in the neck. He touched the patient. He recorded increased breathing, inability to swallow, and drink "returned through the nostrils," (due to paralysis of the soft palate,) and finally death on the fifth day.

His account was so clear that contemporary physicians should be able to diagnose the illness without the use of any modern technology.

Can you? Think for a moment.

Of course it was acute fulminating diphtheria, rarely seen today but common a century ago. Modern medicine is based upon Hippocrates' clinical method of observing, listening, touching, examining, and recording. Here the clinical description took just 78 words, contrasting today's sometimes over-lengthy medical reports.

Hippocrates occasionally noted the patient's environment as part of the tale. For example, in the disease we now call mumps[5] he noted its common season, the climate and wind direction, the population most vulnerable, children and youths at the gymnasium, and its self-limiting nature, thus differentiating it from more serious swellings of the neck or face. One should note that much writing attributed to Hippocrates was likely written by others, for it was the fashion to use a famous name as the author of one's work to give it more authority.[6]

Hippocrates wrote of madness, but little of the influence of the mind in illness, so common in Western society during the past three centuries.[7] Perhaps such cases were less prevalent, or perhaps he was busy with the desperately ill. Sixty percent of the patients he described in Epidemics I and II died.

Today, many patients' problems stem from psychosocial causes, as we shall see.

Vancouver British Columbia, Canada

Dedication

To my family, my patients and other teachers.

Comment

As a clinician who, for 60 years, has been listening to, <u>and hearing</u>, patients' stories, I am in complete agreement with you. In today's hit-and-run managed care medical visit, the art of listening has been replaced by the art of moving the patient on as quickly as possible. Whether we can recover the art of listening is highly problematic.

Edmund D. Pellegrino, MD

Personal correspondence. September 2005

Tales From the Practice

1

LISTENING TO THE RIGHT PERSON

"I'd really appreciate it if you'd come over, Doc, "Harriet's bin to 'arspital 'n' she's no better, 'er breathin's bad."

The voice on the telephone seemed quiet and calm, reflecting her husband's usual manner, yet with a hint of strain. I knew it must be serious; Bob never phoned me about his family's health, something he always left in the capable hands of his wife. Indeed, Bob never visited me about his health if he could help it.

Leaving my office and driving to their home a couple of miles away I thought about the family and Harriet's recent problem. Bob and Harriet had immigrated to Canada from the low-lying Fen district of England and had perhaps naturally gravitated to the low-lying Fraser River delta near Vancouver in British Columbia. They still retained much of their old country accent. They sold eggs and Bob trolled for salmon during the summer.

I had treated Harriet occasionally over the years, delivered their second child and also treated both children for minor problems. Now for five months Harriet had experienced a choking sensation surfacing particularly at night, and she considered her tongue to be swollen. Many times I had questioned and examined her in my office, performed indicated investigations and referred her to an otorhinolaryngologist and an internist-allergist who both suspected allergy but disagreed on possible allergic causes. Removal of allergens and giving medication failed to help. I rather suspected anxiety to be at the root of it, but my listening and questioning failed to produce a solution.

Harriet's symptoms gradually worsened. She feared she would suffocate at night. One evening the previous week while I was away she collapsed at home and was rushed to the local hospital's Emergency department where further examination and tests failed to clarify the problem.

Rain had recently fallen when I crunched up the gravel path toward their home. Roses glistened, chickens pecked, and a black and white mongrel suddenly appeared from behind a wheelbarrow, barked at me, then ran to their front door where Bob appeared. He was a man of medium height, slightly bent in his upper back, broad shouldered and red faced.

"Thanks for comin', Doc...git down, Sophie...don't worry, she's all bark, no bite," he added.

"We've got a dog too," I replied, edging to the right where their living room was. I passed an ancient clock in the narrow hallway, ticking out the time to no-one in particular.

At the far right of the living room lay a plump Harriet, enveloped by a faded blue dress. She was breathing heavily, half propped up with pillows on a window seat, close to the fresh air. I drew up a chair beside her.

Her symptoms were essentially unchanged, her pulse was a little fast but regular, blood pressure, throat, tongue, neck and chest appeared normal. I tried to reassure her that nothing was seriously wrong, but the home visit seemed to have achieved little. I rose from beside her, reaching for my black bag. Bob rose at the same time from an old brown leather chair and accompanied me past the ticking clock to the door. As I reached it he remarked quietly, "May I 'ave a word with you, Doctor?" The rather old fashioned accented phrase eased out half apologetically. "I think I know what's wrong wi' 'arriet."

"You do?" He took an unlit pipe out of his mouth with his right hand and waved the stem in the general direction of the street. "I think it's because of our friends across the road. "'arriet's bin drivin' Karl to 'arspital every day for five month' now; he's nearly blind, yer see - his wife's got cancer, poor soul."

Standing at the front door I heard the whole story, their neighbour's long illness and the delayed diagnosis of pancreatic cancer, the surgery, their hopes for a cure, partial recovery, their hopes dashed, the anxious blind husband usually driven by Harriet sometimes even twice a day to visit his wife in the hospital.

Then came Harriet's increasing concern for them both and her gradual onset of symptoms, of throat tightening and choking. Perhaps she identified with her friend's disease, perhaps it was the regular association with the grieving husband.

For five months my colleagues and I had failed to discover the diagnosis. Bob in his own way had "known" the diagnosis, but had not shared his knowledge with me. The home visit was vital to bring us together in his own environment where he felt comfortable to talk. For Bob and for many patients, hospitals and doctors' offices are foreign, unfamiliar and even frightening territory. Such places may inhibit their natural conversing and providing a full "tale" or "history."

We returned to the living room, sat down and discussed Harriet's illness. At first she was unwilling to accept a psychosocial diagnosis. "Something must be wrong with me," she insisted.

Did she suspect she might have cancer? The fear of cancer is common and could easily develop in her circumstances. Nevertheless, after a long discussion in which she never mentioned any reasonable fear of cancer and after giving her some sedation, I left their home wondering if the visit had been helpful. When I returned two days later she was, to my surprise, considerably improved. Now she wore a brighter dress.After we had talked and I had examined her once more, she walked me to her front door. There was a tennis ball lying on the petal strewn path which I threw for Sophie who chased it and returned in a flash, standing in front of me, tail wagging, soft brown eyes begging for another throw. "If you do that," called Harriet from the doorway, "she'll keep coming back." I turned toward my Volkswagen Beetle. I felt free.

Months later I came across a phrase in New Jersey poet-physician William Carlos Williams' autobiography.

"....I lost myself in the very properties of their minds...." [8]

It would be nice to record that Harriet's symptoms never returned. However, real life medical practice is rarely so tidy. Her breathing improved, but for three or four years she noticed some occasional tongue swelling, a swelling I could never fully substantiate on examination. It no longer troubles her. Despite my diagnostic shortcomings, ten years following the incident Bob and Harriet still choose me as their doctor.

Here is just one tale from among the thousands of visits a doctor makes during his life. I have made more dramatic visits where a patient lay in a pool of blood in the bathroom following a huge gastric haemorrhage or a patient lay in blood-soaked bed clothes following an illegal abortion. But Harriet and Bob's tale well illustrates the potential value of a home visit and of simple listening.

I had followed the usual sequence of history taking and examination in the office, logical laboratory investigation and consultation. Later the patient had made an emergency visit to the local hospital where others tried to solve the problem. None of our efforts helped.

It was her husband who suspected the diagnosis but never shared it with me. To make the diagnosis and to offer logical treatment I had to visit their home, had to spend time listening. Bob had to feel comfortable to offer his diagnosis. It was natural for him to wave his pipe across the road to where blind Karl and his dying wife lived and to suggest the diagnosis.

My treatment was of the simplest kind, listening and discussing. It hardly dignified the important term, "psychotherapy". I was scarcely conscious of treating her. Earlier, as a recent graduate, I might not have accepted the husband's diagnosis. Experience which may bring humility helped. Being busy, I might not have taken the time to listen fully.

Perhaps physicians make fewer house calls today. Most patients can drive to visit their doctors. But, in emergencies, with small children, with the elderly and infirm, home visits may be needed. Meanwhile, the physician can discover clues in his patients' environment. Patients appreciate the effort. In Harriet's case two home visits were economical compared to the previous office visits, investigations, consultations and hospital visit.

A New York neurologist, Dr. Oliver Sacks, confirmed the diagnostic value of a home visit in his marvellous work, <u>The Man Who Mistook his Wife for a Hat</u>.[9] Dr. P, a distinguished musician and teacher, was behaving oddly and failing to recognise people and objects. An ophthalmologist found his vision normal, and, suspecting a deeper problem, referred Dr. P. to Dr. Sacks. As they talked, Dr. Sacks noticed the patient looking at him oddly. Later, while examining him he scratched his left sole to test the reflex. Dr. P. forgot to replace his shoe and even mistook his own foot for it. Considering the examination completed, Dr. P. looked for his hat. "He reached out his hand, and took hold of his wife's head and tried to lift it off." He had mistaken his wife's head for his hat.

Dr.Sacks recounted how he needed time to reflect and then to see the patient in his own environment, i.e. to make a home visit. He arrived with a musical score so they could play the piano and sing together. However, the distinguished musician had lost his ability to read music. Nor could he recognise his family or colleagues in the family photograph album. The home visit allowed Dr. Sacks to further examine his patient's behavior in his natural environment, to discuss the problem with his wife and offer them practical advice. The combined observations suggested a lesion in the brain's visual pathway, likely a tumor.

I am told some doctors never make house calls. They miss a lot.

2

ERIK

Erik walked tall toward my examining room carrying his sixty-nine years effortlessly. Sparse sandy hair arose above a fully lined forehead. His face was slightly flushed, his blue eyes keen and bright and anxious. He seated himself at one end of my examining table, I at the other. "Your blood test's normal," I began.

"Thank God for that," exclaimed Erik with marked emotion and a trace of Norwegian accent.

"I thought when you cancelled my visit yesterday, you needed more time to give me the bad news, that I had leukemia or something."

"Didn't my nurse explain I was just too busy yesterday morning? I didn't want you having to wait...I had two very difficult cases that took unexpectedly long."

"Oh she did indeed, but I didn't really believe her," he added apologetically. "I knew you'd think I'm stupid, but I was terrified I had leukemia."

Norwegian born Erik had emigrated to Canada many years ago. His wife had died young, and he had brought up a family of four children on his own. These were years of working hard, of taking all the responsibility on those broad shoulders, trying to be both father and mother, years ensuring his children had the best education. He had no time to think of himself. Now he was married for the third time. "Grace is wonderful; we are happy together." His open face smiled easily. "We are rich." (He did not mean financially.) "We have nothing to worry about, yet I worry about her and I worry about myself. I keep having these foolish thoughts about my health.

Just since I retired, I had no time before for thoughts like this. Now I've too much time. Oh! I've plenty to do in a way, but I've still more time to think, and I've got more aches and pains than I used to. I'm just getting old, I know that, and I'm more tired than I used to be."

"I understand," I murmured.

"One voice tells me it's all nonsense, imaginary, then another voice suggests it could be leukemia or cancer. The same thoughts come over and over again, buzzing around my head. I know I'm becoming a hypochondriac, but I can't stop these thoughts."

I showed him the actual blood test results, the actual figures. He doesn't know what the figures really mean, but he is reassured by the test result. The test is science, something definite that he can see and believe in.

Now Erik has that off his chest he feels relieved. He brings out a photograph to show me his father's book store back in the old country at the turn of the century.

"I wrote a book a few years back for prospective immigrants coming to Canada from the old country. It didn't sell too well."

"Most books don't," I added feelingly, reflecting on my past experience.

"Well, I mustn't take up any more of your time," he added, rising from the examination table, adjusting his pants and then striding tall out of my office.

Next week he returned.

"I know it's silly, but my stomach's bothering me again. Grace says, "it's just my nerves". If I take those yellow pills of yours, it's better. We call them Dr. Livingston's magic yellow pills. I first took one last

Christmas when I couldn't eat for nausea...and ate a whole Christmas dinner!"

"Let's have a look at your stomach," I replied, slowly feeling over his whole abdomen. There were no lumps, specific tenderness or liver enlargement. "Feels good," I remarked.

"So could I have some more of the yellow pills?" (Actually, stelabid #2).

"Sure get out of the house more, walk five days a week, the weather's fairly good still. Walk more, you'll feel less tired."

He paused.

"I feel I shouldn't be taking up all your time with my foolish little problems; you spend your time in matters of life and death."

"I don't often, you know. Will you try doing some writing again, something creative, try writing some poetry? I would like to see it."

Two weeks later Erik returned to the office. His shoulders were bothering him. I examined them for local tenderness and range of movement. Sitting up on my examination table, he talked mostly about his wife's health. She was short of breath. It was an opportunity also to learn more of his background.

"Tell me about your first wife."

He sighed, turning his head away a little, and then he raised his head.

"No one asks about my first wife. She was my first true love, but she was mentally unbalanced. I loved her, but she spent most of our five years together in institutions. Finally I had to leave her there. I was terribly ill. I was shot by the Gestapo just a day before the end of the war."

"Really?"

"I was in the resistance. We blew up a railway line, and the Gestapo blocked the road. We managed to drive through the barrier, but I was sitting next to the driver and a Gestapo bullet hit me in the chest. Here," he added, unbuttoning a pale blue shirt and pointing to just below his left third rib. I stared at the bullet's small entry scar. Amazing how it missed his heart and major blood vessels. "It lodged in the back of my chest," he added, flipping up the back of his shirt for me to see the irregular scar. "They cut it out, I was very ill for months;

my lungs were damaged. They advised me to immigrate to Canada for my health. I weighed only 108 lbs. There I met my second wife, the mother of my children. She died young, and I brought up the children, did everything for them. I remember ironing my daughter's blouse every morning before school. When all the kids were off to school I left for work."

"You did a marvellous job."

"We read a lot together in the evening. They all went through university."

I could hear the quiet pride and see it in his eyes.

"They used to call me 'the Wizard of Oz', because Dad could do everything. Now they're gone, and I'm retired and I just feel useless."

"That's natural in a way, now you've a lot of time on your hands, but look what you've achieved. You cared for your first wife as much as you could. You fought and nearly died for your country. You raised a fine family. You're still there for them. You've earned their respect and their love. What more can anyone hope to achieve?"

While I was speaking I had moved behind his back and was working on his neck and shoulders with my hands, using massage and traction, those shoulders that have borne so much and now they ache.

Medical corporations underrate its value, Government health schemes fail to understand its importance, insurance companies pay little for it, the profession's bureaucracy takes it for granted, some medical school teachers merely give it lip service, but wise physicians over the years have not neglected it: simple listening.

Erik continued to visit from time to time. His wife, Grace, usually accompanied him. She asked me to listen to her chest. She was short of breath from emphysema in her lungs. It was plain how they loved one another.

Some three years after our first meeting Erik informed me he had coughed up blood for the past week. Strange that he waited a week to consult me about such a significant symptom. Did he fear the cause and wait in hope it would just vanish? I examined his throat and then his neck for enlarged glands and then his chest. I did not have the equipment to fully examine his larynx and sinuses, and suspecting his symptom was serious phoned an otolaryngologist, trying to persuade him to see my patient right away. It is becoming increasingly difficult in British Columbia to obtain specialist help quickly. However, Dr. Wideski saw Erik right away, found a lesion hidden in his naso-pharynx near the base of his tongue, and arranged for a prompt consultation with a cancer specialist.

Strangely enough, the diagnosis eventually proved to be non-Hodgkins lymphoma, not far removed from the leukemia he had feared three years earlier.

After his hospital treatment, Erik and Grace returned to my office to discuss his prognosis. I walked into the waiting room when I heard Brenda, my long-time nurse, chatting with them in her usual friendly way.

"Come into my consulting room for a change of scenery," I said. "You can see the mountains from there."

They sat close together on my old fashioned wooden chairs, Erik tall, sandy haired, straight backed, Grace, darker, more petite, shoulders hunched, strain showing on her face.

Erik leaned forward.

"The Vancouver General was much better than I'd heard," he commented. "I'd heard they were all cold down there, but they were wonderful to me."

"Oh! You would be a good patient," Grace countered.

"But the nurses were so nice to me, they treated me like a king," continued Erik.

"Nurses can make a huge difference," I added.

"And Dr. Wideski, the throat specialist you sent me to, got me seen by the cancer specialist so quickly. I've a lot to be grateful for...."

"I'm so pleased it worked out. Did they tell you more?"

"Not really. I know it's cancer, but somehow I feel better knowing that. You know how depressed I was before. It's so hard to fight that, it's like wrestling with shadows. While I was waiting for the operation it seemed like an eternity. Then it was all over, I think they got it all. The surgeon phoned both Grace, and my daughter. We really appreciated that. When I left, all the nurses came to say Good-bye to me. That was wonderful."

"Did they tell you any more?"

"Not really, just that's it's cancer."

"Actually it's a disease of the blood tissues called lymphoma; it doesn't spread like cancer."

"Oh, that's good."

"It's serious of course, but yours seems to be localised to the back of the tongue. The chest x-ray and other tests are normal."

"Yes, the surgeon said he had never seen anything quite like it before. I believe I'm to go for chemotherapy now. Do you know anything about that?"

"Very little. The drugs are changing all the time."

They both smiled, and then he tilted his head back and began to laugh. Soon we were all laughing together.

I stood up. That seemed a good moment to end the interview.

As he left, Erik turned to me at the door.

"You know, last weekend all my children came down to see me."

"That's pretty special."

Soon Erik started his chemotherapy and suffered from the nausea and fatigue that accompanied it. But he complained little. He was so grateful for the early diagnosis and treatment. In a curious way he seemed to prefer fighting a serious disease, a "real" disease as he put it, than the indefinite thoughts and psychosomatic problems he was experiencing earlier. Indeed his earlier psychosomatic symptoms vanished. He lost his hair and joked about it.

Meanwhile, Grace experienced more shortness of breath from her emphysema. She needed nearly continuous oxygen. I visited them at home as I did not want either of them to pick up infections from other patients who were attending my office. It was a pleasure to see them. They usually offered me a cup of tea or a Norwegian delicacy. We chatted about many things and they showed me their garden.

Gradually, both Erik and Grace improved. Erik was proud of his re-grown hair. Sadly, I retired that summer. I missed them. I could only pass them on to a local family doctor I knew, with whom I thought Erik and Grace would feel comfortable, and who would continue with necessary home visits. I never learned the end of the tale. Perhaps I should have visited them socially, but I felt depressed after ceasing practice and lost my enthusiasm for a while.

Why was Erik ill? His multiple symptoms following retirement signalled anxiety-depression. He was anxious to tell his tale, even more so than Harriet's husband was to tell me their tale. All I had to do was listen. Retirement, which many anticipate so eagerly, often brings health problems, both physical and mental. Existence lost its meaning for Erik and his mind fed upon a vacuum. He could not stop "his thoughts." Interestingly, when his "real" illness appeared, his psychosomatic symptoms were miraculously cured. For now he had something to fight for - his life, and something definite to fight against, - cancer. He found new purpose in living. Such a pattern is not uncommon.

When one listens to a patient with various manifestations of neurotic illness month after month it is easy to drop one's guard and fail to appreciate the seriousness of a new symptom, particularly if it is vague. Of course coughing up blood is obviously a significant physical problem, requiring prompt physical investigation.

Strange how Erik, and many patients and practitioners, have divided illness into serious physical "real" illness and "not serious" psychosomatic illness, while in reality both may be serious and are often closely intertwined.

3

APPENDICITIS

Eleven year-old Larry had had a pain in his belly for a week. Sarah, his mother, brought him to my office and began the tale. She stood by her son who was now lying on the examining table, sweat shirt pulled up, running shorts loose, abdomen exposed. A thermometer placed in his mouth completed the picture.

"I didn't think much of it at first," remarked Sarah. "We all had the stomach flu. Barbara (his sister) had it first, then Larry."

"It's going around," I replied.

There had been a local epidemic of mild gastroenteritis and I had seen a few patients with more severe diarrhoea.

"We got better, Larry seemed better for awhile, but now he's worse again. He was cutting his daily run short, so I knew he must be hurting, and he hasn't eaten a thing."

Larry was training for the school sports. Nothing would stop his enthusiasm. But now he was lying on my examining table not saying much. I retrieved the thermometer, 102 Fahrenheit. His tongue and lips were moist so he was not dehydrated.

"He's been drinking?"

"Some, but no appetite."

"Has the pain changed much, Larry?"

"Can't say, seems all over, like cramps." His face appears slightly flushed, his pulse is fast, 100 beats per minute.

"Have you had a cough or sore throat?"

"No just these cramps and diarrhoea. Oh, and I threw up last night, didn't I mum?" He turns his head toward his mother.

Meanwhile I watch his breathing and how his belly moves as he breathes. Doesn't seem really limited. Now to check his abdomen. My fingers gently feel his upper abdomen, then explore lower down. When they probe deeper on the right side, the belly muscles tighten involuntarily, consistent with appendicitis. The fingers press deeper and then are suddenly lifted away.

Larry takes in a short sharp breath and winces. The rebound test suggests inflammation of the peritoneum, the shiny lining that covers the bowels and the appendix. Next the fingers press deep on the left side and release suddenly. Larry winces again.

"Where does that hurt?"

Larry moves his hand down to the lower right side of his abdomen, verifying the problem is on the right side and is consistent with appendicitis.

Now to check his throat, lymph glands and listen to his chest to make sure he has no problems there and finally to listen to his abdomen for bowel sounds which are present but reduced in quantity.

Why does Larry have pain? It's rather confusing. He seems to have started with gastroenteritis but now has abdominal pain, raised pulse and temperature, distinct local and rebound tenderness in the right lower quadrant of his abdomen. He likely has developed appendicitis, but I've never heard of anyone running while developing appendicitis.

His mother looks on anxiously. She realises it's serious because of the time I'm taking to examine her son.

The office phone jangles. My nurse, Brenda appears at the doorway.

"Sorry to interrupt. Mrs. Freiburg thinks she's in labor; could you speak to her for a moment? It's her third pregnancy."

"I'll just be a minute," I tell Larry and Sarah. Having listened to my maternity patient's description of her five-minute-apart pains, I advise her to go immediately to the hospital and that I'll see her there.

Returning to the examining room, I apologize briefly and say, "I think it's appendicitis, a rather unusual story, but the examination findings suggest it. I've never heard of anyone running when they had it. Larry, you must be tough."   To his mother I add, "I'll phone Dr. Bronson now, he's a good diagnostician and an able surgeon. We'll see if he agrees."

I'm usually fairly confident diagnosing appendicitis. I spent my first year of clinical medicine at St. Thomas' hospital in London. We students all lived in the hospital for a two week period while working continuously at the casualty (emergency) department, existing on four hours sleep a night. Among other cases I saw a dozen acute abdomens, usually in the evening or at night. We students would examine the patient with the houseman. If he considered the case possibly serious, the medical and surgical resident would examine in turn and we students would observe their method of assessment. About 50 percent of cases turned out to be acute appendicitis. We would assist at the operation and be expected to follow the patients later on the wards. I learned more during those two weeks than at any other time in my training. It was hard work, but exciting, and I've enjoyed the challenge of acute abdomens ever since.

Bronson listens to my tale.

"Yes, it's a bit unusual, Mike," he remarks in his gruff voice, "but, it sounds like an appendix. Send them over right away. I'll get him admitted to hospital, have his blood and urine checked, and review him again later. You busy this evening?"

"I've got a mat. patient coming in, so I'll be around." "Oh! I forgot. I didn't do a rectal exam, I knew you'd be doing one anyway. The kid's pretty sick, I didn't think he'd appreciate it being done twice."

"Right. I'll phone you when I've seen the boy."

Returning to my examining room I tell Larry and his mother our plans. "You'll like Dr. Bronson," I added. "He seems a bit formidable at first, but he does very good work."

I used to operate on my own patients with appendicitis and enjoyed doing so. I had done an extra year of surgical training at St. Paul's hospital in Vancouver, B.C. and learned the necessary skills. But fifteen years had passed, and I was seeing many patients with neck and back pain referred by other doctors and I wasn't doing enough surgery to justify continuing it. Actually, with a rather unusual case such as this one I was glad to be able to refer to someone else. I told Larry not to drink anything and then they left for Bronson's office, and a rather irate patient took their place.

"I've waited half-an-hour to see you," he blustered. Heavy set, red faced and impatient he had reason for the increased blood pressure I was monitoring. But I had no time for his attitude.

"Look, I've got a young boy with an acute abdominal emergency. That takes time to assess properly. If he were your son, you'd want him looked after thoroughly wouldn't you?"

"I guess," he muttered.

I examined him swiftly and sent him on his way, still muttering. Then I saw a few patients with minor problems, sore throat, skin rash, sprained ankle, sore back, pap smear, tension headache, bruised thumb, and an insurance form I had to deal with. Then I caught up with a little more of our ever-mounting paper work, made a couple of phone calls and phoned home to tell my wife Diana, I'd be late. "I'll have a bite to eat at the hospital," I added.

Then off to the hospital to check on my maternity patient. Fortunately, she progressed quickly and soon delivered her third daughter. There were no complications and both parents were very pleased. I too was pleased because I had finished the mat case before assisting on a probably infected appendix.

Bronson had obtained an eight o'clock time for the operation, but we were "bumped" by an obstetrician who wanted to do an emergency Caesarean section.

"I'll bet it's no more urgent than our boy," grunted Bronson, a huge man with massive fingers he was now tapping on the telephone book as we sat chatting in the surgeons' room.

"I spend more time sitting on my rear-end than I do operating," he added.

For a moment I wondered about his blood pressure. The operating room was ready by 9:30. Surgical nurse Sheila Dietrich, Bronson and I stood waiting for the anesthetist, sitting at the head of the O.R. table, to put Larry to sleep. He had already started an intravenous in Larry's arm. Now, he injected medication. Larry's bare abdomen was then painted with iodine and surgical drapes were placed in position. Bronson leaned forward, his bulk contrasting the slim youth lying beneath him.

"Knife," he grunted.

Sheila standing at his side slapped the handle of the knife into the palm of his hand and next moment he cut boldly down, exposing the muscle layers in the right lower quadrant of the abdomen and then the shiny peritoneum. Meanwhile I clamped the bleeders as fast as I could. One had to move quickly with Bronson. After the blood vessels were cauterised, Bronson opened the peritoneum more cautiously. Fluid leaked out, slightly turbid with a few little white flakes floating in it.

"Hell, he's got peritonitis," mumbled Bronson, half to himself, and grabbed the culture swab from Sheila who already had it ready for him.

"Retractors!"

He inserted the shiny instruments to expose the area more fully. I must hold them.

"Can't you relax him more, Tony," he asked the anesthetist. The latter busied himself with a syringe to inject a quick acting muscle relaxant into Larry's intravenous. Most surgeons grumble about abdominal muscle relaxation, but anesthetists usually comply to keep them happy.

"Ah! that's better," mumbled Bronson.

"Look at that Sheil," he added to the surgical nurse. Bronson's massive fingers deftly separated the adherent intestines surrounding an angry-looking, engorged appendix with a dirty-looking perforated tip."

"Two inches of trouble," he commented.

Sheila pressed forward to satisfy herself, edging against Bronson in the process. Sheila is attractive and popular with the surgeons, while Bronson enjoyed showing everyone his handiwork.

"I can't believe," I added, "the kid was running while this was happening inside him."

"They likely exaggerated a bit," replied Bronson. "Whoever gives a really accurate story?"

"He's got guts though."

"Yeh! Lots of 'em," responded Bronson, swiftly clamping the base of the appendix, ligating the mesentery and its blood vessels, meanwhile smiling to himself, thinking he had made an apt joke. Then he removed the appendix carefully with a knife and handed it to Sheila.

"Got any saline there, Sheil to irrigate this mess?"

Sheila passed him a bowl full of warm saline and Bronson poured it over the abdominal contents and then suctioned the blood tinged fluid away. Then he made an incision lower down the abdomen to insert a rubber drain, meanwhile remarking, "Don't like drains usually, but I guess one is indicated here." Then he sewed up the tissues in layers, meanwhile asking the anesthetist to give Larry intravenous antibiotics. The whole procedure took just 15 minutes. Bronson was in a hurry to go home, but first he sought out Larry's mother who was waiting at the hospital, so that he could reassure her. Meanwhile, I phoned Diana to hear how it was at the home front and say I'd be back in half-an-hour.

Next day I dropped in to see my maternity patient and a medical case and then Larry. He was in a private room, isolated from the other surgical patients because he was an "infected case." Larry was pale and quiet. An intravenous bottle carried fluids and antibiotics into his arm vein. His mother sat a few feet from him by the window.

"He sure is tough," I remarked to his mother.

"He never was a complainer."

"Dr. Bronson did a great job, but you'll have two or three bad days, Larry, before you are up and around. Your appendix was ruptured. It was a real mess in there."

"I'll give up my running for a couple of days," he responded with a faint smile. His abdomen was tight and I could barely hear any bowel sounds with my stethoscope.

"I'll drop back in a couple of days. Of course Dr. Bronson is looking after you, I'll just come in for a chat."

"We'd enjoy that," his mother replied.

On returning, I find his 17 year-old sister there with his mother.

"You coming in to nurse him,"

"Not me," comments Barbara, " I can't stand blood and stuff."

"How you doing, Larry.?"

"Okay, I guess, but I'm kind of nauseated... the nurse wanted me to eat something," he reported, "but any food makes me sick."

I stood amazed. What eleven year-old needs to be encouraged to eat? I was even more amazed that a surgical nurse would try to encourage a boy with recent peritonitis to eat. Eating might well cause vomiting and even an ileus (paralysis of the bowel).

"What did Dr. Bronson say?"

"He hasn't been in today."

I imagined Bronson would be furious, and I supposed this particular nurse had not had much experience with peritonitis.

"If this was just an ordinary appendix, Larry, you might be eating a little by now, - but, it's not. Forget what this nurse says and just listen to Dr. Bronson."

Listening to his bowel sounds I can hear barely a tinkle.

I think to myself, here's the so-called "team approach" in action. Only one person should make crucial decisions. Today, nursing graduates have more book learning but maybe less practical experience. Nursing and medicine take years to learn.

"It didn't make much sense to me," remarked Larry's mother.

I wanted to lighten the atmosphere so I ask Barbara what she is doing next year. "Think I'll take a year off in Europe and then go to school," she replied.

"You could try medicine or nursing, Larry would give you some practise."

"Didn't I tell you I can't stand blood and stuff?"

Seven more days elapsed before Larry was fit to leave the hospital and six weeks before he could resume running. Next year he came to me with "a bit of a cough." He was running a fever of 103 and I heard some fine râles on the left side of his chest, so I suspected pneumonia which an x-ray confirmed, and I treated him in hospital. I didn't trust Larry at home. He always minimised his problems.

We may also listen to and learn from those who have travelled before us.

Abdominal surgery was avoided in the nineteenth century due to the likely development of peritonitis and death. The immortal Lister, Scotland's precious gift to surgery, who after 1867 struggled to teach others the principles of antisepsis and aseptic surgery, apparently never performed an abdominal operation. [10]

In 1843 Willard Parker [11] of New York drained an appendix abscess, while five years later on the other side of the Atlantic, Hancock,[12] a surgeon to the Charing Cross hospital in London reported opening an abdominal swelling following a long standing ruptured appendix, and letting out the offensive pus. Neither actually removed the appendix.

Singer and Underwood in their <u>Short History of Medicine</u>[13] noted that Rudolph Ulrich Krönlein first actually removed a ruptured appendix in 1886. The patient died. Neither Singer and Underwood in their history [13] nor Talbott[11] in his mentioned Abraham Groves, a Canadian general practitioner/surgeon who had successfully removed a ruptured appendix from a 12 year-old boy in Fergus, Ontario, three years earlier in 1883. [14]

Groves graduated from Toronto Medical School in 1871. He recalled a lecturer in anatomy telling the students that the appendix was an unimportant organ, "because it had no human uses and certainly no diseases." Groves started practice in Fergus, Ontario, near where he lived as a boy.[15] He was 22 years old. By the time he was 25 he had performed his first abdominal operation (May 1874) although he had never seen the abdomen opened during his training. He undertook the operation against the advice of colleagues because the huge ovarian tumor weighing 60 lbs. made life unbearable for the patient. The operation was successful. Before surgery he boiled the water and instruments and washed his hands thoroughly with soap and water. [16] Such practice was unusual at that time. Few believed in asepsis. Lister's teaching was opposed.

Meanwhile, he performed the usual work of a country doctor which involved long horseback rides in all weather as physician, obstetrician, surgeon, friend and counsellor.

In those days appendicitis was commonly called idiopathic

peritonitis and was treated with bed rest and heat or cold applied to the abdomen. In several cases a ruptured appendix would lead to the development of a mass (abscess) in the lower right quadrant of the abdomen. Groves drained some of these abscesses and once saw an inflamed appendix with a perforated tip in the abscess cavity. He reasoned that the appendix was the source of the infection and should be removed at an earlier stage in the illness. On May 10th 1883, he advised an operation on a 12 year-old boy he examined with lower right sided abdominal pain and tenderness.[14]

"On making an opening an inflamed appendix was found. This was removed by first ligating the organ at its origin and also the appendiceal mesentery which was then cut through. The appendiceal stump was sterilised by means of a probe heated in the flame of a lamp..."

The boy did well, but his father was dissatisfied. A neighbour had apparently been treated for the same disease by poulticing and had recovered. The father claimed that no operation was necessary and threatened Dr. Groves. Meanwhile Groves at a later medical meeting found no support among his colleagues for his pioneering method.

In 1887, the renowned surgeon Frederick Treves performed his first appendix operation on a 34 year-old working engineer who had been ill for seven weeks at the London hospital.[17] Treves freed adhesions surrounding the bent appendix, unkinked it, but did not remove it. The obscure Ontario country surgeon had performed a more "state-of-the-art" procedure four years earlier.

Eventually, Groves, who, apart from his regular exhausting work, read widely and contributed extensively to medical literature, developed an enviable local reputation. What a teacher he would have made. He was a class-mate of the great medical teacher, Sir William Osler,[10] but no university offered him an appointment and medical historians[11,13] have ignored him.

How many contemporary students or practitioners have heard of Abraham Groves, the first person to perform an appendectomy for acute appendicitis on the North American continent?

Who has read his 181 page autobiography? A.L. Lockwood in his foreword to Groves' book suggested that Dr. Groves should be included among the "Masters of American surgery."[10] Alas, his work has been forgotten.

Why does the medical profession so ignore its history?

4

A Home Visit Refused

Luka Popovich had a pale olive complexion and a prominent forehead topped with dark hair above brooding, grey eyes. His sensitive fingers were capable of playing the violin, yet strong enough to have strangled two German soldiers when he fought for the Yugoslav resistance during the Second World War.

We met him and his Canadian-born wife Paula at friends of ours over Christmas. Luka was fond of hunting dogs and of bird shooting. An excellent shot, he proudly showed me his engraved shotgun and a rifle when my wife and I visited him during the late spring on their farm in Delta, south of Richmond, close to the Fraser River. Driving up the poplar-lined approach to their farm one could see the solitary giant Mount Baker in the distance overlooking Washington State.

Like many who immigrated from Europe to Canada after the Second World War, Luka was obliged to try his hand at many occupations in order to make a living. Currently he was training hunting dogs, and he offered to train our male Golden retriever Sasha. Sasha, unlike most Goldens, leapt into the water after a duck with all the force of a Chesapeake or a Labrador retriever. Luka loved the dog. He began training Sasha in the early fall.

Soon it was November, and the year was nearing its end. Rain-burdened clouds scudded across the sky, sometimes accompanied by arrows of migrating geese stopping to rest at the mouth of the Fraser River where many commercial fisherman moored their boats at the end of the salmon-fishing season.

Sadly, dark clouds of depression had formed within Luka's sensitive mind. We learned from his friends that he was seeing a psychiatrist. I had no part in his treatment for I was not his doctor. We were just friends or, more accurately, acquaintances.

Early in December, his psychiatrist, Dr. Engels, phoned to ask for my assistance. "Dr. Leevingshton," his guttural voice boomed. "Vould you help me in this deeficult case... You know Luka is very ill. He must be treated in the Mental Hospital."

I replied, "I see," or some other non-committal remark.

"Vould you go to his home and geeve him a strong sedative by injection, chlorpromazine perhaps, triple the normal dose. He has no family doctor. Eef you do this he will be drowsy ven the police come to peeck him up... You are his friend, so vill you do this?"

I hesitated. I had been in solo medical practice for three years, following an assistantship with an excellent medical group in Nanaimo, B.C. so I had had some practical experience and I no longer unhesitatingly obeyed a specialist's request. I also wondered why Luka had consulted a German psychiatrist. He hated Germans.

"Vell, vill you go?"

"I'll go."

All morning I worried as patients came and went. I visited a hospitalised patient in Vancouver at lunch time. While driving, Luka still occupied my mind. If I had been in Luka's place, how would I feel if a friend came and injected me and I woke up next day behind bars in a mental hospital? I would have hated it.

I continued worrying during the afternoon. I walked out of my office, situated in a small shopping centre in South Richmond, and gazed eastward to Mount Baker, isolated beyond the fields. I must go within the hour.

Finally, I made up my mind and phoned the psychiatrist.

"Dr. Engels, I'm sorry I cannot do what you ask. I cannot visit Luka and sedate him." At the other end of the phone there was a pause, then a sigh.

"Very vell."

Christmas came and went. Fresh snow briefly hid the land. Three days after Christmas a distraught Luka knocked at our front door in Richmond. My wife, Diana, home alone with our first child, John, and pregnant with our second, opened the door to a haggard-looking figure, pale faced with sunken eyes. Normally careful of his appearance, Luka wore no tie, and his jacket and collar were askew.

Diana welcomed Luka and invited him to have some lunch. She tried to keep calm. Luka eyed the remains of a turkey on a large dish on the kitchen counter, surrounded by potatoes, brussel sprouts and stuffing. Diana asked him to sit by the counter and placed the turkey, and a plate, knife and fork in front of him. Luka ignored the plate, knife and fork. He tore into the bird with his powerful fingers. His jaws clamped down on the flesh. He swallowed the remaining third of the turkey, the stuffing, the potatoes and the sprouts. Obviously, he hadn't eaten for days.

At last he was satiated, and turning to Diana, he said with a strange dignity.

"Thank you, thank you; I was so hungry."

Then he continued in short bursts exclaiming, "I'm so glad Michael didn't come...the psychiatrist said he would... I was waiting for him with a rifle by the kitchen window...I wasn't going behind bars...I wouldn't let anyone take me...I thought of you, Diana, being pregnant and being left with your young son, but I couldn't let them take me...I watched the drive for his Volkswagen all day... my fingers on the trigger guard, I kept it aimed down the driveway. I felt sorry for you, Diana, but I would have shot him...I wouldn't let them take me...I wouldn't let them take me." His voice trailed off.

Finally Luka left, much to Diana's relief. She phoned me, and I phoned the psychiatrist, wondering what he would do.

Two weeks later we learned that Luka had shot Sasha, the dog he loved, and then himself.

Had I driven up his driveway that December day it is likely Luka would have killed me, for he was an excellent shot. Strangely, I never thought of danger when I refused to make the visit. Perhaps I was naive, but 40 years ago society seemed less violent. Could we have helped Luka?

It is easy to criticise a patient's management, but, physicians face a volume of depressed patients. It is difficult to anticipate who will prove suicidal. Some patients conceal their desire for suicide.

Circumstances may make ideal treatment impossible.

Today, there are newer drugs which, together with listening, help the many of us who from time to time become significantly depressed.

5

CHILDBIRTH ERROR?

Difficult decisions frequently face the doctor as another tale reveals.

Eve lay on her back in the starkness of the delivery room. Her knees were bent, her legs apart, her feet in stirrups. Overhead a ceiling light glared spotlighting her figure upon the central delivery table. A sterile green sheet covered her body.

Bowls, forceps, scissors, syringes and needles glinted from a nearby table. At the head of the delivery table sat the anesthetist, close to the anesthetic machine which was laden with bottles, tubes, gauges and dials. The nurse stood by Eve's side, watchful and waiting.

Eve, near the end of her labour, had made little progress during the past two hours in spite of trying, trying so desperately to push the baby's head down the birth canal. Between contractions she rested quietly, breathing easily. Her pale young face, rounded with pregnancy, was touched with light red blotches. Her lips were dry. She did not complain. She did not even ask how much longer she would be in labour, or whether the baby would be all right.

During each contraction her head twisted from side to side, her dark hair came alive, snaking across the pillow, her facial muscles convulsed, she grimaced, clenched her teeth, and drew her lips back into a tight grin. Her pale face changed to a deep reddish purple, her hands gripped the handles of the delivery table, her knuckles whitened, her shoulders tightened, her back arched, and her lower abdomen and pelvis thrust forward violently. She grunted, she strained and she pushed, and she strained and she pushed, and she pushed...then the spasm left her and she sank back into her own quiet.

The anesthetist asked, "Do you want anything?"

"No, I don't thank you... Oh, I would like a drink of water!"

"I can't give you that, but I'll get you a wet cloth for your lips."

The anesthetist, an understanding woman, brought the wet cloth, and Eve squeezed it between her lips and teeth.

The anaesthetist said, "I'd like to give you oxygen for the baby's sake."

"I don't want it."

"It's not really a drug, and it might help the baby."

"Well, if you're sure it isn't a drug and that it will help the baby, I guess that's all right."

"We really must also give you some medication," I said. "It isn't safe to wait any longer. We must help you get the baby out."

"No, you can't do that. We don't want any drugs or instruments. I've told you already. My husband and I have made a commitment with God. We are in His hands. He'll do what's best for us. We don't want you to do any more."

I thought, How did I get into this mess anyway?' I asked the nurse to have someone phone the administrator and inquire if there should be a consultation. "I can't see what a consultant can do, but the administrator may want one."

Almost immediately another spasm gripped Eve. I sat helplessly before this life and death struggle, this conflict between courage and craziness, faith and stubbornness.

Previously, I had delivered a baby at home for another couple whose religious convictions were incompatible with much of modern medicine. The delivery of their baby, their third, had proceeded quite smoothly, apart from some minor inconvenience to the nurse and myself. I subsequently delivered several babies for members of this religious group who were a kindly people, firmly committed to "natural childbirth." The V.O.N. nurse, Sharon Liske, was enthusiastic about this change from routine and shared with me the duties of waiting, watching and delivering. The deliveries were easy. The husbands would encourage their wives, and children might wander into the bedroom. The women experienced little discomfort and little bleeding after birthing. The oneness of the family was a decided benefit.

I twice refused to deliver a first-born child at home owing to the increased risk.

Eve was not only a member of this group, but was also the pastor's wife. When approached to deliver this baby, their first, I had gently insisted that the birth must take place in hospital. I had said, too, that I would use drugs if they were essential to the welfare of mother or child. I thought they understood.

Eve had a rather narrow pelvis and her baby's head had not turned properly. Her early course in labour seemed long and although no complications had developed, I sensed possible difficulty. Where do these premonitions come from, these feelings of impending tragedy?

I knew I must speak to Eve's pastor husband who was then in the waiting room.

"This birth is taking rather a long time." I said.

"Well, we have every faith in you, doctor."

"Yes, but we may have some difficulty here. Of course I can't be sure, but your wife isn't coming along as quickly as I would like. I may have to use medication to help her in the final stages, and I may well need to use forceps, or even call in another doctor."

"Oh, we don't want that, doctor."

"Don't want what?"

"Drugs or instruments or anything like that. You see, Eve and I have made a commitment with God over our baby. He will look after us. We're in His hands. I'm sure we don't need drugs or anything like that."

"But what if the baby cannot be born without the help of instruments?"

"Oh, we have every confidence in you, doctor."

"That's all very well, but I may have to use instruments."

"You can't."

"What do you mean, I can't."

"I've told you, Eve and I feel safe in His hands. We've made this commitment. Of course, if Eve changes her mind, that's her decision. I believe she'll continue to feel the same way no matter what happens. We don't want instruments or drugs. We're trusting you to carry out our wishes as best you can. I suppose we are being rather a nuisance."

"Well, I don't know what to say to you. Surely you understand that I cannot let either your wife's life or your baby's hang upon your judgment."

"We trust you to fulfil our wishes."

"What if the baby dies?"

"That may be God's will for us. You see, we trust Him absolutely."

I left him. I had never before met anyone quite like him. I felt depressed, irritated, amazed and helpless all at the same time.

Our Father

Who art in heaven

Hallowed be Thy name...

Eve's labour continued while the baby's head descended slowly– so slowly. Eve experienced backache but she never complained. X-rays had confirmed that the baby's head was in a posterior position.

Using tremendous effort Eve strained to push the baby out. She made some progress but her continued efforts would eventually lead to exhaustion. I examined her again and could just determine the posterior position of the head with my fingers pressing into the swollen soft tissues bulging on the surface of the scalp.

Would she be able to deliver this baby? What would happen next? What could I do? They refused consultation with an obstetrician. Should I risk putting on forceps without anesthetic and try to pull the baby out? Could I rotate the head without proper relaxation? Should I force medication against their wishes? What if the baby was damaged following interference by me or a consultant?

The anesthetist and I continued to reason with Eve. She would not change. The anesthetist was very understanding, the nurses were very understanding, the administrator was very understanding.

I sat.

Minutes passed. Push, grunt, relax...push, grunt, relax. The nurse spoke urgently, "I can't hear the baby's heart too well now!" The anesthetist tried to hear. "It seems about 70 and irregular!"

...Thy kingdom come
Thy will be done
On earth...

A little later the anesthetist said, "I can't hear it any more!"

We yell at the woman to push. Eve gives one final desperate push; the head appears at the opening. The baby's hair is dark like Eve's. There is a gush of fluid. I pull and pull. Slowly the head comes down further.

"Suction, quick suction!" I suck out the baby's nose and throat passages for five seconds. Then I pull–forget about tears, forget about everything. Must get this baby out. A shoulder appears, one arm flops out, then the other shoulder, and finally the rest of the baby–a bluish whitish flaccid thing.

It is a little girl.

I quickly clamp the cord and cut it. The anesthetist grabs the baby and rushes her to the incubator and begins resuscitation. She sucks out the baby's air passages with a tube.

Nothing happens. The baby does not breathe. She seems, if anything, bluer than ever. Two minutes pass.

Then the chest makes a fluttering kind of movement; then another. A slight gasping sound escapes and then another. More oxygen, more pressure. A few more gulps. The colour does not change. Three minutes pass. More gulps. Then a deep breath, a rather feeble cry and then another. A pediatrician is present now. But what useful treatment can he offer? Any damage has been done and no-one can repair it. But wait, the baby is breathing a bit more now, the blue colour is changing to a pinkish blue.

The limbs are still limp. The baby looks like a doll plucked out of a ditch by a passing dog.

The mother rests. She feels nothing at first and then relief. We cannot give her the baby. The baby needs oxygen and the warmth of the incubator–she has had sufficient shock.

"Is she all right? Will she be okay?"

"We don't really know yet. We'll have to wait a day or two before we know."

"Thank you so much, doctor. I'm sorry I have been so much trouble."

I could not reply. I felt drained mentally and physically.

All went well for twenty-four hours. The baby appeared to improve steadily. Then she had the convulsion I had been expecting. She was placed on phenobarbital and had no more convulsions. On discharge she looked perfectly well. I tried to persuade the parents to continue the medication at home. They did for a while and then stopped it.

Curiously, the child had no further convulsions. At the six week check-up, both baby and mother were doing well. The parents were grateful, almost pathetically grateful.

...For Thine is the kingdom
And the power
And the glory...

I could not analyse my feelings. I was relieved that we had apparently escaped a major tragedy. I was still very disturbed by this case, feeling I had been forced to practice poor obstetrics. At the same time I partly admired the courage of these people in a society where personal sacrifice is increasingly rare. I knew I had not heard the last of this case from the hospital. One of the protections that the public has towards reasonable medical standards is the hospital "rounds." During "rounds" unusual cases or cases with management problems are presented. Rounds also provide opportunities for education.

The public never sees this side of medical care and some people imagine that doctors always cover up each other's mistakes. Actually, rounds can be a humiliating experience for the unfortunate physician. Some doctors relish dissecting their colleagues and demolishing their management of a case. Not only do some specialists enjoy attacking general practitioners but also one another.

I expected criticism and got it. Rounds next week began in a small lecture room with a discussion of my unusual case. The resident in obstetrics stood up in front of the room and described the details of the case. I then moved by shaking legs to the front of the room and began to speak. I sensed a state of rising tension in the room. My stomach tightened as I tried to describe my difficulties. I finished and sat down.

Up jumped a young obstetrician. He was a super expert, having just completed his speciality training three months earlier and having therefore a full three months career in obstetrics behind him.

"In all my experience," he proclaimed pompously, "I have never come across a worse managed case. It is difficult to understand how any doctor practising obstetrics could refrain from taking the elementary precaution of having a consultation. Of course I would have put on forceps at once and delivered the baby. This is a case of gross mismanagement." An instant expert, he ranted on for some time about what should or should not have been done. I felt more stupid than ever.

A pediatrician then sprang to the attack. He briefly criticised my work and then continued, "Of course Dr. Livingston should have notified the coroner. The baby should have been made a ward of the court and the parents sued on behalf of the baby." One or two others rose to the attack and finally the Chief of Obstetrics pronounced, "If these people did not want proper medical care, they should have been put out on the street and had the child in the gutter!"

I thought, Semmelweis of Vienna or Hippocrates of Cos would have wondered at that statement. What rubbish! Here we are advancing steadily into the sixteenth century. These doctors want to punish someone, either me or these simple, earnest people. I could almost hear a priest saying, "Recant and your soul will be saved and we can take you off the rack!" The inquisition had been resurrected. Heresy must be stamped out at all costs.

...Forgive us our trespasses
As we forgive them who trespass against us...

At last two people came to my defence. The anesthetist kindly said that she felt it was a very difficult case and I had done all I could. Then an obstetrician I did not know rose and added a spark of humour to the darkening scene. "Of course I wouldn't have handled the case like Dr. Livingston – not me! I would not have called in a consultant no, I would have called in at least two consultants–anything to shift the responsibility to someone else! Life's too short to make heroic stands for people. It's impossible to look after patients like these."

Silently I thanked him. He did not know me. I had never referred patients to him. Maybe he felt that he should support the underdog. He came from a religious background that is usually considered a minority. My stomach untied itself. It had been a memorable forty minutes. I left for the day's work exhausted but relieved. At least they hadn't thrown me off the staff. I decided not to accept any more patients from this group. We are not often so lucky twice.

But the case did not end there. The hospital obtained independent opinions from two highly respected legal firms. Opinion, as so often among lawyers, was divided. One firm suggested I should have notified the coroner, should have obtained a consultation, should have applied forceps and should have delivered the baby. The other suggested I should have proceeded in the way that I did and that to interfere further could have been interpreted as assault.

Seven years later I was reminded of the case when a woman approached me on a ferry and said, "It's good to see you after all these years, doctor."

I tried to remember. I have difficulty remembering names, but I did realise she was a friend of Eve's.

"How are the pastor and his wife and the little girl?"

"They're fine."

For Thine is the kingdom
And the power
And the glory
For ever and ever....

Perhaps I should add that the case of the pastor and his wife occurred over 40 years ago. Close fetal monitoring was unavailable at the time. Today, under similar circumstance, consultation would be mandatory.

Obstetrics remains a challenging art. Insurance costs and other social factors discourage many family doctors from broadening their experience to include this usually pleasurable task, perform a valuable service and lessen the fracturing of health care. Despite occasional moments of terror, obstetrics remains one human activity where patient's trust develops, vital to effective health care.

6

No Time To Listen

Richmond, British Columbia, where I spent most of my medical life, lies at the mouth of the Fraser river delta on Canada's west coast, just above the U.S./Canada border. The delta harbours flocks of migrating geese and ducks which fly in during the evening to feed on farmers' fields. Now, it also harbours a large population of people.

In the fifties, Richmond was primarily agricultural, where vegetables, strawberries, and feed for cattle were harvested. Sadly, the rich delta soil, richest farmland in Canada, soon became covered with housing, a questionable policy. My patients, mostly Canadian born or immigrants from Britain or Europe, lived in those homes.

In the late spring, the Fraser River slowly rises, fed by melting snows of mountain ranges. The rate of common infective illnesses and depression following the long winter also rises. One April week, heavy laden clouds hovered as patients filled the office suffering mostly routine problems. Life was dull. Then someone new phoned and the voice sounded urgent to my nurse-secretary Fran.

"I've just put my back out, I'm passing through Vancouver today. Could I see the doctor? I hear he's good at backs."

Fran who shared nursing duties with Brenda, fitted the new patient into the afternoon schedule. He arrived walking gingerly, six foot four inches, tilted to one side and supported by a cane. He was black. Mahood Luonga leaned against the waiting room wall until I was able to examine him a few minutes later. He removed his jacket and shirt slowly, the movement causing obvious discomfort. We eyed each other, standing by the examining table. He was muscular and in perfect condition. He smiled easily, his ever-so-white teeth contrasting his ebony skin. Later I learned he was an African visitor, son of a tribal chief, who was studying for his doctorate in political science at Berkeley in California. However, his physique resembled that of a tight-end for the San Francisco Forty-Niners.

"It's silly really," he remarked. "I just leaned forward to lift a suitcase out of the trunk of the car we'd hired and felt something snap in my back."

"A common story," I replied, "Let me check your back before you lie down. I'll ask a few questions as we go. Would you turn around and loosen your belt?"

He moved slowly and faced away from me, partly tilted to the left.

"Put your finger on the sorest spot."

He placed his index finger just to the left of his fifth lumbar vertebra.

"Bend forward as far as you can easily."

He bent slowly about 15 degrees, then stopped.

"And backward."

He did so more easily. I placed my fingers on the crest of his pelvis to check the level on each side.

"Try bending to each side."

He is more restricted bending to his right.

"Now, lie down on the examining table."

Cautiously, he complied.

"Have you ever had a similar pain before?"

"No."

"Does it move anywhere?"

"No. - Oh! I guess my left buttock aches."

"Any serious illnesses in the past?"

"Had malaria a few years ago, but nothing recently."

"Any accidents?"

"A rear-ender on the freeway two years ago."

"Any symptoms?"

"Sore neck for a few days."

"Treatment?"

"No, just took a few aspirin."

"What position helps your back?"

"Lying with my legs bent."

"And your worst?"

"Sitting."

"Coughing make it worse?"

"Haven't coughed."

"Taking any medication regularly?"

"No," he replied with a smile, "I don't like pills."

"Any allergies?"

"No."

I could have asked Mahood more questions about his weight, urogenital system, bowels and so on, but obviously he has a mechanical back problem. He just wants his back fixed. I've other patients to see and a limited time in which to examine him. All I really need to do is to rule out a prolapsed intervertebral disc. So I tested his ankle and knee reflexes and the strength of his ankle movement, up and down against resistance. All were normal. I tested his straight leg raising and found it limited 10 degrees on the right side and 40 degrees on the left. Straight leg raising on the right side did not cause pain on the left side. (The crossed straight-leg raising test.) If straight leg raising had been more limited on both sides, and if straight leg raising on the right side had caused significant pain on the left, the patient might have had a prolapsed intervertebral disc. Likely, in addition, there would have been changes in one of the reflexes or weakness of the ankle movement.

My neurological examination was limited, but it covered the essentials. Next, I asked Mahood to lie on his stomach and I palpated the tender area in his lower back, partly to see how much muscle spasm was present, and how he responded to pressure, and indeed because patients expect to have their sorest spot examined. Thoroughness breeds confidence.

I asked him to roll over onto his back once more.

"I know your back hurts, but I don't believe it's serious. I won't send you for x-rays. They are unlikely to help, and it would mean driving to an x-ray facility, more sitting, lying on a hard table and driving back here again. You have mechanical back pain. It's not a disc problem. Probably one of your facet joints is locked low down on your left side. I think I can help by trying to unlock it with my hands. Any questions?"

"No, it would be great to have it fixed. I have to fly out of here by nine tonight."

"I'll give you a prescription for Tylenol threes later; that's Tylenol with some codeine. Take two every three to four hours for a couple of days, and then only if you need it. Drink enough water when you swallow them. Also I'll show you two simple exercises to help stretch your back before you leave. Now, roll over on your right side."

Mahood eases over. I moved to the other side of the examining table facing him. Then grasped his left ankle and gently bent his knee and thigh three times back and forth. Next, I leaned over him, placed my right arm and hand across the crest of his pelvis, digging my fingers just right of his first sacral spine. Then I placed my left arm over his bent left thigh and left pelvic crest, fingers just to the left of the spine of his 5th lumbar vertebra. I asked Mahood to breathe slowly in and slowly out, meanwhile taking up the slack in the tissues between the fingers of my two hands and thrust with my left hand upward and to the left, causing a sudden slight distraction of the vertebrae, my left forearm helping as a lever. There was a slight popping sound from his back and a grunt from Mahood. I asked him to roll over onto his back and bent his thighs back on his abdomen a couple of times while his knees were bent.

Then I asked him to stand up. He complied, and, cautiously at first, began to move his back forward and backward and from side to side. He was soon moving easier and his tilt had lessened. Gradually, his black face widened with a smile revealing ever-so-white teeth.

"I never thought," he exclaimed! "I'd find our kind of treatment over here!"

Evidently, my manipulation was similar to that performed by his tribal healer. I shared in his pleasure. Such a dramatic response occurs occasionally.

Then I showed him a simple deep breathing and rocking exercise he could do while lying, an exercise that has been passed down through the ages. I also showed him how to bend backward while standing with his thumbs digging into his lower back.

"While you are flying this evening, walk round the aircraft every 20 minutes or so and stretch, to prevent your back stiffening again."

I was most interested in the history of manipulative treatment in different countries. Standing before me was the son of an African chief who likely would have known his tribe's history and the work of his tribal healer or witch doctor. Obviously, I would spend the next few minutes questioning him. Possibly, here was the chance of a lifetime to learn something of the history and origins of manipulative treatment.

But I had spent 25 minutes with him, the office was now bulging with patients, and I was captivated by Mahood's pleasure and his radiant smile. The idea of questioning him further did not occur to me until after he had left the office. Then, as if a blow had struck, I realised what an idiot I had been, and I had no way of contacting him again.

Ah! those missed opportunities.

Few medical doctors use manipulation in treating their patients' backs, necks, shoulders or other body parts. Medical schools teach students little physical medicine and even less about spinal manipulation. Nor do these schools consider the omission important. Patients however, flock to manipulators of different stripes, consulting osteopathic physicians, chiropractors, some physiotherapists who have learned manipulative techniques, or unlicensed manipulators. Chiropractors term the procedure I performed on Mahood, "the million dollar roll."

Massage and manipulation are two of the oldest remedies known to man. We should not be surprised to learn that Hippocrates, whose work we considered in the introduction, used manipulative techniques. Concerning manipulating the spine he recommended: [18]

"The physician, or some person who is strong and not uninstructed, should apply the palm of one hand to the hump, and then, lay the other hand upon the former and press, attending to whether this force should be applied directly downward, or toward the head or toward the hips." Here he advised manipulating the spine according to the patient's functional anatomy, the planes of the facet joints.

Hippocrates also treated some patients with spinal deformities by "succussion," in which patients were suspended upside down and shaken upon a ladder. However, he warned, "I have been ashamed to treat all such cases in this way, because such modes of procedure are usually practised by charlatans." [19]

Dr. James Cyriax included a photograph of a two thousand year old statue from a Buddhist temple in Bangkok, Thailand, in his Textbook of Orthopaedic Medicine.[20] The statue showed manipulation of the lower back.

The famous Iranian physician, Avicenna, (979-1037), reproduced illustrations of Hippocrates's methods of traction and pressure on the spine, while the father of French Surgery, Ambrose Paré (1510-1590) used and wrote about spinal manipulation. Captain Cook, suffering from sciatica during one of his voyages, was squeezed by Tahitian women in 1777. In his diary he noted how they "cracked" his bones.

In Europe, certain families were known as bone setters, Knochenbrechers, (Germany), Les Rebouteux, (France), or Kotknackare (Scandinavia), the name developing from the belief that they could put a bone back in place. They had no formal education, but passed their knowledge to their children, for bonesetting was a valuable trade.

Sarah Mapp, also called cross-eyed Sally, developed a reputation for bonesetting and unorthodox behaviour in Epsom, UK, about 1736. Some described her as an ignorant, drunken savage, but a popular song was more generous.

"You Surgeons of London who puzzle your pates,
To ride in your coaches and purchase estates;
Give over for shame, for your pride has a fall,

The doctress of Epsom has outdone you all."

In 1831, John Eberle at Ohio Medical college proposed that the spine could be the source of some illnesses, writing,

"When the pains are situated in the head and upper extremities, the spinal affection, if any exist, will be found in the cervical vertebrae; and when a part about the chest, and upper portion of the abdomen, is the seat of the painful affection, there will probably be spinal irritation in one or more of the dorsal vertebrae." [21]

Hugh Owen Thomas, the father of British orthopaedic surgery, descended from a family of bonesetters; but, seeing severe damage caused by bonesetters manipulating tuberculous bones and joints, became a strong advocate of rest. Nevertheless, having suffered a skeletal pain for many years he consulted the renowned bonesetter, Hutton, and was "instantly relieved" of pain.

Sir James Paget, a celebrated surgeon, advocated learning from bonesetters when he delivered a classic lecture on "Cases that bonesetters cure," to staff and students at St. Bartholomew's hospital in London.

He stated that,

"The patients who are cured never cease to boast of their wisdom in acting contrary to authorised advice; but they who are damaged are ashamed of themselves and hold their tongues...for the patient loves to be cured with a wonder, and the audacious confidence of these conjurors is truly wonderful."

A canny Scot, he added,

"Few of you will practise without having a bonesetter for an enemy. And if he can cure a case which you have failed to cure his fortune will be made and yours marred."

Finally he advised his listeners,

"Learn then to imitate what is good and avoid what is bad in the practice of bonesetters...."

His words drifted through the lecture theatre and were later published in the British Medical Journal in 1867,[22] only to be ignored by the medical profession to this day.

Dr. James Mennell of St. Thomas' hospital, London, his son John, Dr. James Cyriax and Janet Travell, physician to President John

Kennedy, were more recent medical advocates of manipulation as one valued form of therapy, encouraging physicians, especially general practitioners, and physiotherapists to learn the simple skills necessary. Sadly, few physicians responded.

Meanwhile, non-physicians followed the bonesetters. Andrew Still, a civil war soldier and healer who lost three children to meningitis, founded osteopathy about 1874 and likely influenced Daniel Palmer who founded chiropractic (Greek, Kheir, hand and Praktikos, practitioner) about 1895. His enthusiastic son B.J. Palmer developed chiropractic into a flourishing business.

Spinal manipulation sparked my interest in a curious way. During the sixties I used to attend weekly educational lectures at St. Vincent's hospital in Vancouver. One morning a well-built local orthopedic surgeon, Dr. Gerald Burke, was demonstrating the techniques of spinal manipulation. He asked for a volunteer among the doctors present. No one seemed eager to step forward. I was somewhat sleepy at 8.00 a.m. having seen a patient the previous night and drowsily volunteered.

Gerald Burke soon cured my drowsiness. A powerful man, he enveloped my head in his arm and rotated it violently while I sat in a chair. There was a loud crack, associated with slight discomfort. Then he turned it in the opposite direction. Having experienced the first procedure I involuntarily resisted the second and experienced more discomfort. I should add that I had no symptoms or neck problems at the time. However, I developed a mild headache for the next couple of days. Afterward, I wondered about the treatment. Presumably, it must help someone. Medical school and internship had given me little helpful instruction in managing the common problem of backache and neck pain. Maybe manipulation could be one useful tool. At least I would investigate it. Burke generously invited me to see his work twice a week for a couple of hours and instructed me in his methods which he had learned in the United States.

He saw a huge volume of referred patients whom he swiftly assessed and treated. I tried to hear the patients' tales before Dr. Burke assessed them, and then after treatment follow them up at a later visit.

In four weeks I became reasonably competent in manipulating patients' lower backs, mid backs and necks. Hesitatingly, I tried these methods in my own practice using rather less force and less rotation, and found that I was able to help some patients whom I had previously been unable to help. No patient appeared to suffer significant injury in Burke's hands nor in my inexperienced hands. I was somewhat concerned over Burke's quick assessment and felt he might miss some less common but serious problems.

Later that year our family visited Ireland where my wife's parents then lived, and I took the opportunity to visit Dr. James Cyriax at St. Thomas' hospital in London, England. A little balding, enthusiastic man, he assessed patients very thoroughly. He and his physiotherapists instructed me in their methods. Like Burke he was a powerful manipulator. Later, he kindly replied to my queries briefly on postcards. (Considered unorthodox by other staff members, Cyriax was visited by many physicians.)

I was introduced to Dr. John Mennell in Los Angeles. He graciously invited me to stay for a couple of days. I learned from him and from Dr. Janet Travell and attended some meetings of their North American Association of Manual Medicine. I approached an osteopathic teacher in Los Angeles, Dr. John Andrews, and learned his gentle techniques. Later through a local physiotherapist, John Oldham, I saw Norwegian physiotherapist Freddie Kaltenborn's and New Zealander Robin Mackenzie's approach to patients. Over the next few years local doctors, who at first were suspicious of my new interest, began to refer their patients. Most were general practitioners and I felt honoured to see their patients. When Dr. Bill Sutherland, chief of surgery and teacher at Shaughnessy Hospital in Vancouver, started sending me a few neck and back patients, I realised I must be doing something right.

I continued to read widely but was always concerned about possible injury. Therefore, I kept careful notes on patients treated, and also asked patients if they experienced any ill-effects following manipulation from any source. Over a three year period, May 15, 1966 to May 15 1969, I questioned 676 consecutive patients and eventually gave a paper on the subject to the North American Association of Manual Medicine.Dr. Janet Travell, President John Kennedy's doctor, was impressed by the paper. She commented, "You must prepare your paper for publication and submit it. I will write to the editor of <u>Clinical Orthopedics</u>, and he will publish it."

In due course <u>Clinical Orthopedics</u> published it.[23] A few months later I was walking up the stairs of Vancouver's courthouse to give evidence in a traffic injury case when I met Dr. Arthur McConkey coming the other way. McConkey was chief of orthopedic surgery at St. Paul's hospital in Vancouver when I completed a year's residency in general surgery including orthopedics.

We smiled vaguely as we passed. Suddenly, he roared, "Livingston!" I turned to face him, "How the hell did you ever get into <u>Clinical Orthopedics</u>?"

"Well, - it was a reasonable paper, wasn't it?"

"Sure, but how did you get in there?"

I smiled, he smiled. Then we went our separate ways. I didn't like to tell him of Dr. Travell's letter to the editor. Of course, McConkey knew that quality journals such as <u>Clinical Orthopedics</u> rarely published papers from obscure general practitioners. Medicine has its caste system.

Why have so few medical doctors investigated spinal manipulation, used for hundreds of years in different cultures to this day and easy to learn? Why does modern medicine with all its advances neglect such a common area of pain. Mahood Luonga and thousands like him often do not find the most appropriate treatment in a medical doctor's office.

Generally speaking, medical leaders have rejected chiropractic as their ancestors rejected bone-setting.[22] Meanwhile, chiropractors with their hands-on emphasis have achieved some patients' trust and had their treatment covered by worker's compensation and insurance companies. In 1992, Drs Curtis and Bove from Chapel Hill, NC, recommended physicians refer their back patients to chiropractors.[24] However, in a series of letters replying to their article, physicians from five communities pointed out chiropractic irregularities such as treating diabetes and meningitis, and advising heart failure patients to discontinue essential medication.[25,26] Meanwhile neck manipulation continues to cause some strokes and neuropathy.[27,28] Physicians contemplating referral to a chiropractor should visit that specific chiropractor to see the methods and scope of his practice. The physician should also understand "the entire range of chiropractic therapeutic claims." [25]Official studies on the effectiveness of spinal manipulation suffer from design weakness. Surely the most effective researcher is history. Patients have sought manipulators for centuries and appreciate a physician who uses manipulative skills when indicated. Eight years since retirement I still receive occasional requests from people with spinal or shoulder problems to treat them. One recent person did so during the 2004 Athens Olympics, - some 2400 years after the great physician Hippocrates taught manipulative methods in Greece.[18]

Returning once more to my practice, I employed manipulation for 35 years as one useful tool in mechanical back and neck pain associated with limited movement. I never caused a significant injury. The vast majority of cases were referred by other practitioners. In addition, I taught basic manipulative principles for ten years. As time passed, I began to see more referred patients with difficult pain problems where the chief cause was not always mechanical. To find the cause invariably meant paying more attention to patients' tales. I also began to see patients referred with so-called "whiplash injury."

7

THE WHIPLASH MYSTERY: TALES NOT TOLD

If an occupant of a car struck from behind by another vehicle experiences a sore neck and related symptoms such as headache or dizziness within 48 hours of the accident it is reasonable to consider the symptoms are due to the accident. The occupant has suffered a sprained neck, commonly referred to as a "whiplash injury."

One would expect such a sprain to improve within six weeks as do other sprains which people experience such as ankle sprains. Indeed, Martin, a specialist in physical medicine at the Mayo Clinic, stated in 1959 that the vast majority of whiplash patients should improve within six weeks.[29] In 1994, Barnsley, Lord and Bogduk agreed,

"The usual expectation would be that sprains or tears of muscle would heal in a matter of weeks, forming a scar within the muscle but leaving the patient with no residual pain."[30]

Why then do some patients continue with their symptoms and disability long after six weeks?

First, let us consider the tale that is not told, illustrated by four narratives.

Case One:

Many years ago an insurance company asked me to assess a 35-year-old woman who had been injured in a moderate impact car accident four months earlier and still experienced pain in her upper back and chest following considerable assessment and therapy. Maria had red hair and pale skin. She appeared tense and irritated, perhaps thinking of me as "the insurance doctor," and my being the fifth doctor asked to examine her.

I asked her all the appropriate questions. There were no unusual features to her accident. Examination disclosed mild local tenderness, a full range of movement in her neck and back and normal neurological findings. I was dissatisfied at the end of the consultation and asked her to return so I could recheck her findings and so we would have the opportunity to talk together more.

The second visit did not seem to be accomplishing anything. I was tired after visiting a patient during the night and finally could think of nothing more to ask. We looked at each other across my office desk. Seconds ticked by. Tension slowly built. A full minute passed.

Suddenly she burst out, "My mother had a pain like this. In three months she was just skin and bones."

Hesitatingly, she described her mother's battle with cancer. Daily she saw her mother suffer from back and chest pain caused by bone cancer. Daily she saw her flesh disappear. Daily she witnessed her misery. When her own pain did not improve following her visits to the doctors and more visits to the physiotherapist, she began to fear she had cancer. Fear multiplied her pain.

Fear of cancer is common, as Sarno, a New York specialist in physical medicine, pointed out in a 1981 article.[31] It is often unexpressed. In chapter one, Harriet never expressed fear of cancer. Many folk believe that a blow can "turn into" cancer. I must emphasize that I discovered her fear, the cause of her persisting symptoms, not by some clever technique, or by asking questions, but by not asking a question, by saying and doing nothing.

Many years ago Michael Balint, a psychiatrist at London's Tavistock Clinic, described how ineffective asking patients many questions can be.

"In essence medical history-taking means collecting answers to our well-tried set of questions. More often than not, practically everything else that the patient tries to tell his doctor is pushed aside as irrelevant."[32]

"Our experience has invariably been that, if the doctor asks questions in the manner of medical history-taking, he will always get answers- but hardly anything more. (My underlining) Before he can arrive at what we called 'deeper diagnosis,' he has to learn to listen."[33]

On the other side of the Atlantic in Rutherford, New Jersey, poet-physician William Carlos Williams in his autobiography had written earlier of the patient's deeper diagnosis.

"My business, aside from the mere physical diagnosis, is to make a different sort of diagnosis concerning them as individuals...."

He summed up the practice of medicine and of poetry as a "lifetime of careful listening."[34] Maria was not my patient. But I was able to reassure her to some extent and suggest to the insurance company that they send a copy of my report to her family doctor.

Case Two:
Forty-three year old Tanya also illustrates how significant past events affect our response to an accident. Her lawyer referred her to me for a medical-legal opinion a year after her accident. Tanya related the following tale.

She was the driver of a then stationary car struck from behind by another vehicle. At impact she was facing ahead. The impact threw her head violently onto the dashboard. Nevertheless, she experienced no initial symptoms.

It was not until five days later while typing at work that suddenly she felt the whole right side of her body go numb, from the top of her head to her toes. Later she experienced headaches and pain between her shoulder blades, and in her right arm and leg.

Two family doctors, an orthopedic surgeon and two physiotherapists treated her without any apparent improvement. The surgeon had prescribed exercises after diagnosing a sprain between her shoulder blades.

Tanya's symptoms were unusual. First, after a severe blow to the head one might have expected headache or other symptoms within 48 hours. There were none. Her first symptom, sudden numbness over the complete right side of her body occurred after a space of five days. Such one-sided total numbness is unusual after a whiplash injury and suggests the possibility of a psychological cause such as hysteria. Yet, when I digested a copy of the orthopedic surgeon's report, there was little information about her past medical history, merely, "she gives no history of having had similar previous complaints." There was no note whatsoever concerning her family history. These omissions surprised me, considering the character and length of symptoms and the failure of all physical treatment to date.

Perhaps the secret of her pain lay in the past. To fill in the gaps I asked Tanya about her previous health and about her family life. It didn't take long. Soon the flood-gates opened and she poured forth details of her tragic past. Her mother used to beat her regularly with a poker when she was a child, to the extent of driving her down onto the floor with repeated blows. This battering continued until Tanya grew old enough to resist.

Years later, by a curious twist of fate, her mother and her father both suffered strokes, and her mother whom she particularly hated became paralysed down the right side of her body. Currently Tanya was separated from her husband and was supporting her two sons. When she developed sudden numbness on the right side of her body she became obsessed with the thought that she might become paralysed and would not be able to work any more. She had repressed the memory of her childhood violence for many years; but now, the accident and her demanding responsibilities had triggered her bizarre symptoms.

Tanya's lawyer naturally expected that my examination would strengthen his case. However, when my report reached him, revealing the multiple reasons for her symptoms, he phoned me pretty fast.

"Are you sure you're correct?" he queried.

"Yes."

"It seems weird to me."

"You're a lawyer, not a doctor. This is a classic case of conversion hysteria-right out of the textbook. She wouldn't be having her symptoms without her accident; but neither would she be having them without her tragic past."

He grunted his dissatisfaction and immediately shunted her off to a psychologist and a neurologist for their opinions. The insurance company lawyer countered by obtaining two opinions from his experts.

Apparently two of the four experts agreed with my diagnosis of conversion hysteria and two did not. In any event, I doubt if being forced to visit all the doctors helped Tanya who merely became a pawn between doctors and lawyers.

I never learned the end of the tale. Tanya's case must have been decided out of court, for I was not called to give evidence. I hope that when the legal action was finished, she was able to resume her life.

Frequently, consultants in whiplash cases do not obtain essential details of a patient's past health and life because the patient does not wish to give them, or feels they are irrelevant, or the consultant does not spend time listening for them. Usually, consultants have just one visit in which to assess a patient and may fail to see the whole picture. The next tale illustrates similar points.

Case Three:
An insurance company asked me to assess a middle-aged woman 14 months after her front-end collision. (For space reasons I will make a few minor non-essential changes and omissions.)

Mary stated she was the front-seat passenger in a pick-up which struck a car broadside. The impact caused less than a thousand dollars damage to her pick-up, suggesting it was moderate. Three days later her neck stiffened. Pain in her neck, right shoulder and arm followed. She visited a chiropractor who at the time was treating her lower back, then a family doctor whom she hardly knew. He advised rest and anti-inflammatory medication which bothered her stomach as she had had prior "stomach ulcer trouble".

Four months later she changed doctors. She was referred to a rehabilitation specialist. A CT scan showed a "bulging disc," a finding that worried her. Changing doctors again she was referred to a neurosurgeon whose report I read and who considered the CT scan suggested a C5/C6 herniated disc. However, his examination findings did not appear to support that diagnosis. Mary consulted a lawyer one month after the accident who advised her to keep a daily diary. She continued diarizing for the next six months. Currently she was not working.

She had had a previous motor vehicle accident followed by low back pain and two years of chiropractic treatments. Also she had had a stomach ulcer, past family troubles and a hysterectomy and bladder repair. She denied having neck pain prior to the accident or current family problems.

Multiple factors might have delayed her recovery, and I noted "unknown social factors" as one possibility in my report summary. I spent time showing Mary half-a-dozen exercises she could do three times a day to help herself and gave her illustrative sheets to show her doctor for his approval. Finally I advised a limit to passive treatment, part-time work within four weeks and reassessment within two months if she was not working regularly.

Mary's experience is repeated time and again in minor whiplash injuries.

Unfortunately, nearly a year passed before the insurance company requested reassessment. However, the company now provided the full case file including the invaluable case notes of the doctors and chiropractors during the six years prior to the accident.

The consultants' reports were essentially similar, although the rehabilitation specialist and a neurologist considered the problem to be merely a soft tissue injury, while the neurosurgeon suggested the possibility of a protruded cervical disc. Interestingly, these specialists gave very little information concerning the patient's past or family health.

For example, the neurologist stated, "In the past she has had a history of sciatica and she has had a previous complete hysterectomy. She has no allergies."

He did not mention the prior accident, the prior chiropractic treatment, nor any family history. Neither the neurologist, rehabilitation specialist or neurosurgeon mentioned that the patient kept a diary, describing her symptoms <u>every day for six months</u>, surely a vital fact.

None of us obtained a prior history of neck pain. Both the neurologist and the rehabilitation specialist honestly commented, that given the type of accident, it was difficult to understand how her symptoms could have persisted.

Interestingly, the diagnosis lay all the time not in the consultations by the experts but in the regular case notes of the family doctors and brief records of two chiropractors. Chiropractor X noted that Mary had presented with neck pain in 1988, 1989 and 1990. Chiropractor Y's one line note in 1993 was "C1-C2 S1+3," and in 1994, "C4 and +3," presumably indicating symptoms from or therapy to these cervical segments. The records, brief as they were, suggested pre-existing neck pain treated prior to the accident, pain she had denied.

Meanwhile, during the six years prior to her accident Mary had consulted family doctors because of "recurrent bladder infections," "tendinitis of the left elbow," "pain on intercourse," "abdominal pain referred to her back," "cramps and gas," "enlarged bowel due to constipation," "pressure feeling in her bladder," " wax in ears," "a lump" (not stated where), "sore spots on labia," (new partner denies having herpes,) "sore throats" etc. The list is very similar to patients' complaints lists given in Michael Balint's book, <u>The Doctor, His Patient and the Illness</u>.[35]

Usually she preferred visiting chiropractors for her neck or back complaints. However, following her current accident she did report neck and back pains to her family doctors and remarkably, for 18 months following her accident there is no record of any of her old or other multiple symptoms. They were entirely replaced by neck or back symptoms. Experienced family doctors observe such patterns quite commonly.

To sum up, Mary suffered from multiple symptoms mostly due to chronic neurotic illness. The accident simply became a new focus for her problems. Her medical legal case was settled soon after the lawyers digested my second report explaining the situation.

Much time, effort and money, visits to doctors, chiropractor, physiotherapist, massage therapist, lawyer and insurance personnel were wasted because the tale was not told.

Case four:

This was more complex. A Professor of Dentistry referred 50 year-old Gloria to me for assessment and treatment of persisting pain. Injured three years earlier in a motor vehicle accident, she described it dramatically,

"It felt like an earthquake, tremendous noise. I imagined the car completely accordionised. I was frightened, the door wouldn't open, I couldn't get out, I imagined the gas tank could explode...."

She developed dizziness, pain in her head, neck, shoulders, upper back and visual symptoms. She lost concentration and memory, and could neither work nor do much at home. She visited a family doctor she had seen only once before, then many specialists, other health practitioners including physiotherapists over 100 times, a pain clinic, a rehabilitation centre and a psychiatrist. Finally, the insurance company had her see their orthopedic surgeon and psychiatrist. She criticised some practitioners but admitted her rudeness to them. The insurance company's psychiatrist scared her so she never told him her full story. (I knew him to be a most reasonable person.) Meanwhile, the psychiatrist she liked refused to continue treatment until the medical-legal aspects of the case were settled. She thoroughly disliked her lawyer, and relations with her husband were deteriorating.

I realised this case was a disaster, and after examining her briefly and teaching her some exercises, suggested she return next week when she could spend as much time as she liked. In the meanwhile I wanted to discuss her with her family doctor who had wondered initially about the possibility of a psychological cause but had followed usual medical practice by referring her first to physically inclined consultants.

On the next visit Gloria told me of repeated scary dreams in which she was trapped, "she was running but not moving." At times she became terrified in their car and started screaming. She had flashbacks of the accident. Then she described a little man who kept following her. "He moves so fast you can't see him." Obviously she had paranoia. Finally, she described her son's tragic death following a head injury in a motor bike accident. She remained with him while he lay for a week in a coma. She had encouraged him to buy the motor bike hence suffered from sadness and guilt.

Examining her a second time I found consistent limited neck movement and limited turning of her upper back to the left. Placing her hands behind and between her shoulders was limited. Neurological examination was normal. To me her problems were both physical and mental. She appeared to have post traumatic stress syndrome, a diagnosis also favoured by her family doctor.

I used manipulation and taught her exercises to help restore neck, shoulder and upper back movement, and I used listening to help her anxiety-depression. On another visit I asked her to draw a picture while seated at my desk. From a group of coloured crayons she chose a black one to reproduce the view from my window. She depicted the worker's compensation building tilted at a sharp angle as if it were falling, and a road with a little red car on it and two trees, one of which appeared to have a face within its foliage. I asked her if the car and the trees meant anything to her. She replied that the car was the one that hit her, while there was a face in the tree, the man who had been following her.

The picture suggested fear, depression and paranoia. I wished she was still seeing the psychiatrist and discussed her problem further with her family doctor. In view of Gloria's experiences with psychiatrists we decided we would both support her and avoid further referrals unless she worsened. Meanwhile Gloria had started volunteer work at an old people's home which seemed a positive sign.

Over the next six months her symptoms, mood and range of movement began to improve. I urged Gloria not to go to court but to accept the insurance company's offer. I doubted whether her story or attitude would impress a judge. However she insisted.

The judge was not impressed with her or with my evidence, preferring naturally enough the psychiatrist's opinion, for he had an excellent reputation and frequently gave evidence in court. The psychiatrist rejected the diagnosis of post traumatic stress syndrome. As Gloria had been trapped in a traumatic accident, had suffered immediate terror, later symptoms including depression, flashbacks of the accident, screamed occasionally in their car, and had repeated scary dreams of being trapped and being unable to move, I thought the diagnosis reasonable.

However, she had omitted most details when she visited the insurance company's psychiatrist because he scared her. In short, the tale was not told, or as Australian psychiatrist J. Ellard put it, "there are many things in heaven and earth that do not emerge in a psychiatric interview."[36]

To conclude Gloria's case, the judge nevertheless allowed her reasonable compensation. I never learned the end of the tale for I was unable to contact Gloria after the case was settled. Nor did she return to her family doctor – an all too familiar pattern.

Generally speaking it is wise to check the medical literature to see if others have reported similar cases. Actually I could find few articles with case reports revealing the presence of psychosocial factors in whiplash injury cases. Describing and publishing such case histories seemed no longer fashionable.

In 1964, a psychiatrist, James Hodge,[37] described four cases in Ohio similar to the ones already described. I will summarise them briefly.

A 43 year-old white woman whose stationary car was struck from behind, lost consciousness and awoke in hospital complaining of pain in her neck and shoulders. An orthopedist asked Dr. Hodge to see her two weeks later for "nervousness." She did not complain to him of pain, but of crying for no reason and fear of being alone, or that something was "going to happen." Hodge treated her with interviews after a Sodium Amytal injection which helped her to tell her full story and relieved her symptoms. Then she began to reenact the accident in her dreams. He could find no underlying psychosocial problems.

His second case was a 33 year-old white woman passenger hit while in a car struck unexpectedly from behind. She developed intermittent nausea and faintness, pain in her neck and shoulders and difficulty swallowing. She became nervous, afraid to drive in a car and easily fatigued. She occasionally dreamed of someone being hit by a car. She had been "nervous" all her life, especially after her father had experienced concussion following a car accident from which he had never fully recovered. He felt that "something was draining from his head into his chest." She also was treated with narcosynthesis and spoke of her fear of a "cancer in the neck, and nobody will tell me," and of her fear of injury or death. She was reassured.

The third patient retained symptoms of pain in the head, neck and back, plus numbness and partial loss of function in her left arm, none of which could be explained organically. She gave a long history of personal maladjustment and psychosomatic problems. During treatment it became clear that she handled life's stresses by developing psychosomatic symptoms.

The fourth case involved a young woman with a mild whiplash injury who stated that she had been "nervous" since the death of her grandfather eleven years previously. It demonstrated a similar pattern to the others.

In Canada, Andrew Malleson reported a similar type of case in 1990.[38] Peter, a 28 year-old unmarried history teacher had six years previously been apparently injured in a rear-end collision without vehicle damage. He had complained of continuous neck and back pain ever since which failed to respond to "various innumerable treatments." "A host of medical experts" had provided evidence for and against his damage suit. He had had a domineering alcoholic successful lawyer father and a submissive mother. He had experienced anxiety episodes while standing in front of his class in the past. Such attacks had produced chest pain and he had visited a hospital emergency department. He was a loner. Now he was incapacitated, dependent and emotionally repressed. Malleson, noting that Peter had wasted six years of his life in this fashion, asked, "Can physicians and the law make compensation litigation less dangerous for others?"

While we cannot generalise on so few cases, we can note repeated parallel findings. For example, eight out of the nine described patients had a long history of neurotic illness. Seeing multiple practitioners proved ineffective, while experts did not consistently obtain past and family histories wherein lay the secret. Invariably, physical treatment was preferred before psychological assessment. Physical problems sometimes coexisted with psychological ones. Changing physicians and differing opinions muddled some patients. Communication between practitioners and others was sometimes lacking.

Today, we are dazzled by new technologies in medical care. However our cases suggest that we fail to understand people. Formal history-taking is not sufficient. Practitioners must learn to listen more.

Interestingly, Farbman reported similar findings in the Journal of the American Medical Association in 1973.[39] He studied 136 patients with uncomplicated neck sprain to investigate the great disparity in duration of symptoms and contributing factors not directly related to the injury. He found that the four most significant factors delaying recovery were emotional factors, extensive medical history, overtreatment and litigation.

Reviewing the cases of Maria, Tanya, Mary and Gloria confirms Farbman's observations.[39] Medical students are taught to refer their problem patients to experts, who, it is assumed, will assess patients thoroughly and obtain the correct diagnosis.

These four anecdotal reports suggest that assumption may not be accurate, particularly in cases where psychosocial factors are present. All patients were referred to specialists, usually multiple specialists, and received considerable therapy. Their accidents were considered to be the cause of their symptoms despite limited history-taking,[32,34] and the failure of physical therapy. In Mary's instance, family doctors actually had clues to the likely cause of her pain in their case records revealing previous multiple visits for psychosocial problems. Gloria's doctor had considered a psychosocial cause for her symptoms but, programmed by her training, kept referring Gloria for physical assessment and treatment for a full year. Gloria's case was more difficult to assess because she had abnormal physical findings of limited neck and shoulder movement which required appropriate physical therapy as well as managing her psychosocial problems. Many patients' symptoms have both a physical and a psychosocial origin. We need physicians and therapists who are trained to appreciate that both physical and psychosocial factors may be present in the diagnosis. About 20 years ago I gave a lecture on whiplash to a branch of the Insurance Corporation of British Columbia. At the conclusion there was a free-for-all discussion in which an experienced elderly insurance agent commented wisely.

"I listen to them," he remarked quietly, "they tell me about their lives. The vast majority who continue to have symptoms and continue to have treatment are unhappy or confused people living in difficult circumstances."

By careful listening he frequently discovered "the tale that had not been told," and had come to comprehend what many experts and many researchers have not.

However, insurance companies usually consider accidents from a purely mechanical view. They take little notice of an adjuster or physician who balances mechanical with psychosocial factors. "Whiplash" conferences demonstrate such bias.

Companies might find it more helpful and less costly to provide their staff with personal copies of Listening in Medicine and my 1999 work Common Whiplash Injury, Charles Thomas.

8

PARALLELS

In the past century modern medicine's success was based upon the earlier pathological, physiological and public health contributions of Rudolph Virchow[40] and others. Their work attributed a specific cause to a specific illness and led to medicine's emphasis upon specificity.

Appalled by the living conditions of the majority and the high incidence of diarrhoea among infants, Virchow investigated sewage disposal and water supply between 1862 and 1872. After much research he introduced a new sewage disposal system into Berlin[41] and reduced infant mortality dramatically.

We should note that Virchow held not only a specific concept of illness, but also a much broader social one. Earlier, in 1848, after investigating a typhus epidemic in Silesia, he had concluded that "poor sanitation, ignorance of basic hygiene, lack of education, and near starvation were the root problems of the epidemic."[42] Concentrating upon one specific cause for an illness, most medical teachers have relatively ignored social causes of illness which were Virchow's lifelong concern.

Social causes of illness find parallels with our tales. Hippocrates[4,5] had considered the patient's environment as one possible cause for illness, while in chapters one and two psychosocial factors were prominent in both Harriet's and Eric's illnesses. In chapters three, five and six, the problems of appendicitis, childbirth and mechanical back pain all seemed entirely physical, yet all revealed social aspects. The "whiplash" cases reported in chapter seven seemed to be mechanical problems at first; however the real cause of persisting symptoms was psychosocial, and the patients failed to improve because psychosocial factors went unrecognised. Multiple consultations and tests, particularly well demonstrated in the cases of Mary and of Peter did not help; rather, they prolonged the problem, just as repeated consultations and tests failed to help Harriet's difficult breathing in chapter one. The secret path to diagnosis lay in taking time for careful listening.

Further parallels can be seen from the work of Michael Balint. In the 1950s, he, together with a group of general practitioners in London, UK, studied the difficult cases in their practices – patients who did not improve despite much investigation and treatment. Invariably, Balint and his co-workers found the hidden causes of the illnesses to be chiefly psychosocial and the commonly used medical diagnostic methods futile.[43]

Balint described how patients "offered" an illness and then he commented upon the physicians' responses.[44] As for conventional history-taking in which the doctor asks the patient his "well-tried set of questions," and often "pushes aside as irrelevant what the patient tries to tell him," Balint commented that the doctor will get answers, "but hardly anything more."[33] The important matters may be the "irrelevant ones"[32] the patient was trying to tell him.

Furthermore, doctors live with the fear that they might miss something. That something is commonly thought to be a hidden physical problem. However, they rarely fear missing psychosocial problems which may affect patients just as much and sometimes even more than physical illness. Doctors are conditioned by their training to consider all possible physical causes first.[45] Diseases are, in effect, given a "ranking order" of importance,[46] as are the patients who have them. Doctors prefer to diagnose physical disorders which they feel more comfortable managing. Furthermore, patients whose complaints may be traced back to demonstrable or assumable anatomical or physiological changes rank higher, and patients with psychosocial problems are in a way the "dregs left over...."[46]

Doctors are trained to eliminate inappropriate diagnoses by a series of physical examinations.[47] It is assumed incorrectly that the patient's attitude to his illness is unchanged by this series of examinations.[47] It is also assumed incorrectly that finding a negative result and reassuring the patient that "nothing is seriously wrong" will invariably help the patient. Often it does not.[43,48]

Rheumatologist Nortin Hadler pointed out the dangers of the diagnostic process in his work, Occupational Musculoskeletal Disorders. People feeling out-of-sorts for longer than usual may consult a physician after starting their own diagnostic process. Not uncommonly after examining the patient, "nothing" is found, but, "diagnostic uncertainty furrows the brow of the physician and is rapidly taken to heart by the patient."[49] Soon, "physician and patient join in the hunt for a diagnostic label.... Blood is drawn, and imaging studies scheduled. The patient leaves the office a changed person." As the patient waits for the test results to trickle in his worries and fantasies increase. Soon he is medicalised.

Furthermore, to interrupt the diagnostic process by now suggesting psychosocial reasons for the symptoms may well engender patient hostility.[50] Already the patient has been programmed toward believing in a physical cause for his symptoms, and psychological illness is stigmatising in America.[31,50]

When a doctor, uncertain how to best help his patient, requests a consultation from a specialist he tends to regard the latter as an authority, rather as he did his teachers in medical school. However, in cases where the diagnosis has a strong psychosocial element it is often difficult to decide upon an appropriate specialist, for many specialists have had little training in psychological medicine and indeed may know less about the subject than the referring doctor. Consultants are experts in their specific field but may "pretend to know more than they actually do."[51]

In "whiplash" cases the problem of referral is difficult. For example, if a practitioner requests a neurologist to see his patient he expects a thorough history taken, a full neurological examination to be done and a relevant report provided. But, as we saw in Mary's case (chapter seven), such a thorough assessment is not always made. Here the neurologist took an inadequate history, merely stating, "In the past she has had a history of sciatica and she has had a previous complete hysterectomy. She has no allergies." He failed to mention the prior accident, prior chiropractic treatment, and family history, or the fact that the patient kept a daily diary, recording her symptoms every day, a <u>process that naturally leads to symptom retention</u>. He performed a thorough neurological examination, but surely that was only one half of the assessment.

Incidentally, family doctors are influenced by their consultants' reports, and may place less importance upon patients' histories because some consultants obviously do so. In a 1998 editorial in the <u>Journal of the Royal Society of Medicine</u>, Fleetcroft deplored the decline of the general physician (general internist) and that current consultants concentrated increasingly upon their specialties and often did not offer patients a full assessment and diagnosis.[52] Also he noted that in difficult cases it may not be clear which specialist is most appropriate. Referring to an inappropriate consultant frequently results in the patient "being shuttled" from one specialty to another, "having lengthy and ill-judged investigations with no consultant taking overall responsibility."[52] One can see this "shuttling" effect in the cases of Tanya and Peter in chapter seven.

Balint noted that the commonest cause of dissatisfaction among general practitioners concerning consultation was that "consultants gave opinions and futile pseudo-pyschiatric advice on a sorely inadequate basis instead of stating squarely and sincerely that they found no illness belonging to their special field which would account for the patient's complaints...."[51]

Reviewing the patients' tales in chapters one to seven we can find many parallels to Balint's research,[32] a work that has been available to doctors and others for over forty years, but in North America seems to have been ignored.

Patients may provide just part of their tale during their first visit to a new practitioner. If a patient learns to trust that practitioner he may add further material during subsequent visits. Such "obtaining a history in bits" is familiar to experienced general practitioner/family doctors and can be well seen in chapters one and two and in cases two, three and four in chapter seven. Naturally, people are less likely to expose their secrets, weaknesses and follies to doctors they hardly know. Therefore, it is very difficult for consultants during one visit to understand the whole person who is consulting them. Even astute psychiatrists can be led astray, as was seen in the case of Gloria in chapter seven. Indeed, many patients object to being referred to a psychiatrist, particularly in whiplash cases.

There is a further parallel. Our case reports confirm Sarno's observation on the common fear of cancer.[31] Harriet in chapter one and Eric in chapter two were two examples. Ironically, Eric later did develop a type of cancer. Two of the whiplash cases in chapter seven, Maria and Dr. Hodges' second reported case revealed a hidden fear of cancer. Such a fear is likely to increase following unhelpful tests and treatment. Furthermore, that fear may generate still further symptoms.

Some authorities and medical editors may eschew the tales or research we have considered as being "merely anecdotal" and having little or no serious scientific value. I suggest that repeated experiences are indeed valid, and have increased authority when confirmed by other observers. Readers can decide for themselves whether or not the more complete case histories reported here or those reported by Dr. Oliver Sacks in The <u>Man Who Mistook his Wife for a Hat</u>[53] are sometimes the only way to adequately describe a problem and are worthy of being considered valid research.

Concerning whiplash injury, we will consider further parallels toward the end of the book.[54] Meanwhile we will listen to the past and explore the importance of the tale or case description to previous general-practitioner-observers.

Many of their experiences parallel ours. They achieved much with little technology. Some learned the value of listening.

Listening to the Past

Just as the tale of the patient is neglected in medical training, so too is the history of medicine, thus narrowing students' vision. Most of these tales should also interest general readers.

9

EDWARD JENNER (1749-1823)

Why? is the question the child asks. Why? is the question the researcher asks. Students in the health sciences are given a massive amount of information. There is hardly time to ask "why?" Edward Jenner, born in Gloucestershire, England in 1749, was one student who asked why.

For centuries smallpox had been a fearfully contagious and often fatal disease. Macaulay in his <u>History of England</u> described it thus,[55]

"And smallpox was always present, filling the churchyard with corpses, tormenting with constant fear all whom it had not yet stricken, leaving on those whose lives were spared, the hideous traces of its power, turning the babe into a changeling at which the mother shuddered, making the eyes and cheeks of the betrothed maiden objects of horror to the lover...."

Young Jenner was an apprentice to a Gloucestershire surgeon named Ludlow. With Mr. Ludlow he saw a patient named George Perkins who had developed the fearful disease. Nevertheless, a dairymaid named Ann volunteered to nurse him.[56,57,58]

"Have you had smallpox or been inoculated with it?" Mr. Ludlow asked her.

"No sir," she replied. "I cannot take it for I have had the cowpox. I have nursed several persons and have not come down with it."

Jenner was astonished that she would fearlessly expose herself to the dread disease. Was it really true that persons who had developed cowpox could not develop smallpox? While Mr. Ludlow dismissed her remarks as mere superstition, Jenner was not fully satisfied with that explanation.

Indeed a popular ballad of the day ran as follows,

"Where are you going my pretty maid?
I'm going a milking, Sir," she said.
"What is your fortune, my pretty maid?
My face is my fortune, Sir," she said.

Popular tradition was telling science that milkmaids who commonly would have developed cowpox would not suffer the ravages of smallpox.

The seed idea of a relationship between small pox and cowpox began to form within Jenner's mind. Meanwhile other matters commanded his attention. He trained for a short time under the renowned surgeon and anatomist John Hunter from whom no doubt he learned some research principles.

After starting his own practice in the Gloucestershire countryside, Jenner continued a correspondence with Hunter who asked him to work on specimens brought back from one of Captain Cook's voyages. As a child, Jenner's interest in natural history had led him to collect fossils. Now he investigated salmon, described how the newly hatched cuckoo pushed a hedge sparrow out of its nest, postulated on the migration of birds and noted the temperature of hedgehogs. In 1775 Hunter wrote to Jenner:

"I thank you for your experiment with the hedgehog; but why do you ask me a question by way of solving it? I think your solution is just; but why think, why not try the experiment?"

Meanwhile the young doctor continued his country practice

which involved the hazards of epidemics, clinical problems and riding through inclement weather.

"The ground was deeply covered with snow, and it blew a hurricane...half of my face and my neck was for a time wrapped in ice...I had the same sensation as if I had drunk a considerable quantity of wine or brandy...my hands at last grew painful...when I came to the house I was unable to dismount without assistance. I was almost senseless...." Also he continued his medical investigations, being among the first to describe Angina Pectoris in 1778 and heart disease following rheumatism in 1789. Jenner's broad interests included building a huge balloon with friends and flying it from Berkeley Castle. He was fortunate to find a wife who sympathized with his interests.

His research experience helped when Jenner turned to think once more about smallpox and its possible relationship with cowpox. First, he had to find and describe cases of cowpox. Finding cases was an immediate problem because those who developed the mild disease rarely consulted doctors about it. He cross-examined patients and friends to see if they ever had had the two diseases. Next, he inoculated with smallpox some farm workers in whom he had personally observed cowpox. He obtained the material from the smallpox hospital in the city of Gloucester. All held the country belief that those who had had cowpox would not develop smallpox and allowed him to inoculate them. None became ill.

One month later he rode to Alveston with his notebooks to attend the first autumn meeting of the County medical society. He presented his findings with enthusiasm only to encounter chilly silence. When he suggested inoculating humans with cowpox to prevent smallpox the other doctors just laughed at him.

One surgeon declared, "To say that cowpox and smallpox are related is to imply that animals and humans are of the same family. The sacrilegious nature of such an allegation is only too clear. I have grave doubts of a colleague's competence who is willing to clothe the superstitions of milkers with the mantle of scientific investigation."

Another doctor insisted that "he be sternly rebuked and warned not to pursue his researches further on pain of being expelled from the society."

There were reasons for their opinions, for while smallpox

inoculation had been tried and was sometimes effective, in a number of other patients it had actually caused the disease.

Jenner rode back to his practice the next day depressed by the violent reaction to his work and that no one would help him. Only Mr. Ludlow stood by him.

During the next few years he continued his practice and his observations on nature. Then suddenly smallpox broke out in his district. People were terrified. Jenner and other doctors were forced to inoculate with smallpox despite the risk. He was unable to test his theory that cowpox inoculation would prevent smallpox for there was no cowpox material available. He inoculated his own baby with swinepox, a disease that looked similar to cowpox. Later he inoculated his baby with smallpox. There was no reaction.

Then, despite the opposition to his preventive use of cowpox, his experiences had so convinced him of its potential value against the deadly smallpox that he decided to "try the experiment". On May 14, 1796, he inoculated an eight year old boy with cowpox material taken from a dairy maid. The boy developed cowpox. Six weeks later Jenner inoculated him with smallpox. There was no reaction.

"I selected a healthy boy (James Phipps) about eight years old, for the purpose of inoculation for the cowpox. The matter was taken from a sore on the hand of a dairy-maid (Sarah Nelmes), who was infected by her master's cows, and was inserted on the 14th day of May, 1796, into the arm of the boy by means of two superficial incisions, barely penetrating the cutis, each about half an inch long.

On the seventh day he complained of uneasiness in the axilla, and on the ninth day he became a little chilly, lost his appetite and had a slight headache. During the whole of this day he was perceptibly indisposed and spent the night with some degree of restlessness, but on the day following he was perfectly well. In order to ascertain whether the boy, after feeling so light an affection of the system from the cowpox virus, was secure from the contagion of the smallpox, he was inoculated on the first of July following, with variolous matter, immediately taken from a pustule. Several slight punctures and incisions were made on both of his arms, and the matter was carefully inserted, but no disease followed."[59]

On July 19, the country doctor wrote to a friend Edward Gardiner, "I have at length accomplished what I have been so long waiting for."

Two years later he completed his manuscript on An Inquiry into the Causes and Effects of the Variolae Vaccinae.[59] Sixty-four pages long, it cost seven shillings and sixpence and was published twenty-seven years after he had first wondered at the connection between cowpox and smallpox while an apprentice to Mr. Ludlow.

Before his book was published, he travelled to London with his wife and daughter and tried to interest the doctors in the value of cowpox inoculation. Although introduced by the wife of John Hunter he met continual scepticism and unwillingness to try his cowpox material. The doctors knew the dangers of injecting smallpox and simply doubted that an obscure country doctor could come up with a remedy that had eluded experts for years. William Woodville, Chief of the London Smallpox Hospital, told him it was "nonsense".

Finally, after four months of rejection, tramping London's cobbled streets, and using up his savings, he left London for the more peaceful countryside. Just before leaving he happened to visit a surgeon, Henry Cline, who had also studied under John Hunter. Cline later tried one of Jenner's quills of cowpox on a patient with hip disease at St. Thomas' hospital, thinking it might prove useful as a counter-irritant.

After inoculating his patient with Jenner's cowpox material, he inoculated him later with smallpox material in three places. There was no reaction. On August 9, 1798 he wrote to the country doctor,

"...I think the substituting of cowpox poison for the smallpox promises to be one of the greatest improvements that has ever been made in medicine. The more I think on the subject the more I am impressed with its importance.

With great esteem, I am, dear sir

Your faithful servant

Henry Cline."

Cline's successful test confirming Jenner's experiments followed the publication of The Inquiry. The two events stirred the nation. The Inquiry became a best seller and requests for the vaccine poured in from all parts of the country. Cline wrote to Jenner that if he were to open a practice in London he could be assured of ten thousand pounds yearly

- a fortune. The country doctor replied simply, "...Shall I who, even in the morning of my days, sought the lowly and sequestered paths of life – the valley, and not the mountain – shall I, now my evening is fast approaching, hold myself up as an object for fortune and for fame? What stock should I add to my little fund of happiness?

My future, with what flows in from my profession is sufficient to gratify my wishes; indeed, so limited is my ambition, and that of my nearest connections, that were I precluded from further practice I should be enabled to obtain all I want.

As for fame, what is it? A gilded butt, forever pierced with the arrows of malignancy."

Some still resisted the country doctor's discovery including Woodville, the smallpox expert who, trying to repeat the experiment merely "cleaned his instruments off with a cloth," his poor technique actually transmitting smallpox by mistake. By 1799 the battle was nearly over when 33 leading London doctors published their agreement with his discovery. Soon his life-saving material spread around the world and persons such as Catherine, Empress of Russia, Napoleon Bonaparte and Thomas Jefferson recognized the country doctor's extraordinary contribution. Jenner's material was later replaced by weakened smallpox vaccine. His discovery was the first major step in our preventive immunisation for such killer diseases as smallpox, diphtheria and polio. When you take your children to your doctor or nurse for their immunisation, remember the country doctor.

And, remember Ann, the dairymaid who first intrigued young Jenner with her crucial tale.

10

HUNTINGTON'S CHOREA

Medical research does not always lead to a cure, but careful case description is always valuable.

As a youngster, George Huntington, (1850-1916,) used to accompany his physician father as he visited his patients in East Hampton, Long Island. One day as they drove down the rough road by horse and carriage, they passed two women, mother and daughter, gesticulating wildly, walking erratically and grimacing. George was astonished by their antics and questioned his father about them.

His father knew of the family although they were not his patients. George learned that they suffered from a rare disease which was known fearfully as "that disorder" by the afflicted families. The disease was passed down though the generations, becoming apparent in early adulthood.

George's fascination with the disorder continued when he became a doctor. He learned all he could find about the disease noting its clinical and familial features and searched through the records of his father and grandfather.

Later, on February 15, 1872 he described his findings at a medical meeting in Middleport, Ohio,[60] beginning his paper with a general description of chorea or St. Vitus dance as commonly seen in children. He noted the cause was unknown but it sometimes led to inflammatory heart disease.

He described chorea as a disease of the nervous system. "The name chorea is given to the disease on account of the dancing propensities of those who are affected by it, and it is a very appropriate designation. The disease, as it is commonly seen, is by no means a dangerous or serious affection, however distressing it may be to the one suffering from it, or to his friends. Its most marked and characteristic feature is a clonic spasm affecting the voluntary muscles. There is no loss of sense or of volition attending these contractions, as there is in epilepsy; the will is there, but its power to perform is deficient. The desired movements are after a manner performed, but there seems to exist some hidden power, something that is playing tricks, as it were, upon the will, and in a measure thwarting and perverting its designs; and after the will has ceased to exert its power in any given direction, taking things into its own hands, and keeping the poor victim in a continual jigger as long as he remains awake, generally, though not always, granting a respite during sleep. The disease commonly begins by slight twitchings in the muscles of the face, which gradually increase in violence and variety. The eyelids are kept winking, the brows are corrugated, and then elevated, the nose is screwed first to the one side and then to the other, and the mouth is drawn in various directions, giving the patient the most ludicrous appearance imaginable. The upper extremities may be the first affected, or both simultaneously. All the voluntary muscles are liable to be affected, those of the face rarely being exempted...."

Then he continued by describing a rare form of the disease which occurred almost exclusively on the east end of Long Island and which he called hereditary chorea.[60]

"The hereditary chorea, as I shall call it, is confined to certain and fortunately a few families, and has been transmitted to them, an heirloom from generations away back in the dim past. It is spoken of by those in whose veins the seeds of the disease are known to exist, with a kind of horror, and not at all alluded to except through dire necessity, when it is mentioned as 'that disorder.' It is attended generally by all the symptoms of common chorea, only in an aggravated degree, hardly ever manifesting itself until adult or middle life, and then coming on gradually but surely, increasing by degrees, and often occupying years in its development, until the hapless sufferer is but a quivering wreck of his former self.

It is as common and is indeed, I believe, more common among men than women, while I am not aware that season has any influence in the matter. There are three marked peculiarities in this disease:

1. Its hereditary nature.
2. A tendency to insanity and suicide.
3. Its manifesting itself as a grave disease only in adult life.

1. Of its hereditary nature. When either or both the parents have shown manifestations of the disease, and more especially when these manifestations have been of a serious nature, one or more of the offspring almost invariably suffer from the disease if they live to adult age. But if by any chance these children go through life without it, the thread is broken and the grandchildren and great-grandchildren of the original shakers may rest assured that they are free from the disease. This you will perceive differs from the general laws of so-called hereditary diseases, as for instance in phthisis, or syphilis, when one generation may enjoy entire immunity from their dread ravages, and yet in another you find them cropping out in all their hideousness. Unstable and whimsical as the disease may be in other respects, in this it is firm, it never skips a generation to again manifest itself in another; once having yielded its claims, it never regains them. In all the families, or nearly all in which the choreic taint exists, the nervous temperament greatly preponderates, and in my grandfather's and father's experience, which conjointly cover a period of 78 years, nervous excitement in a marked degree almost invariably attends upon every disease these people may suffer from, although they may not when in health be over nervous.

2. The tendency to insanity, and sometimes that form of insanity which leads to suicide, is marked. I know of several instances of

suicide of people suffering from this form of chorea, or who belonged to families in which the disease existed. As the disease progresses the mind becomes more or less impaired, in many amounting to insanity, while in others mind and body both gradually fail until death relieves them of their sufferings. At present I know of two married men, whose wives are living, and who are constantly making love to some young lady, not seeming to be aware that there is any impropriety in it. They are suffering from chorea to such an extent that they can hardly walk and would be thought, by a stranger, to be intoxicated. They are men of about 50 years of age, but never let an opportunity to flirt with a girl go past unimproved. The effect is ridiculous in the extreme.

3. Its third peculiarity is its coming on, at least as a grave disease, only in adult life. I do not know of a single case that has shown any marked signs of chorea before the age of thirty or forty years, while those who pass the fortieth year without symptoms of the disease, are seldom attacked. It begins as an ordinary chorea might begin, by the irregular and spasmodic action of certain muscles, as of the face, arms, etc. These movements gradually increase, when muscles hitherto unaffected take on the spasmodic action, until every muscle in the body becomes affected (excepting the involuntary ones) and the poor patient presents a spectacle which is anything but pleasing to witness. I have never known a recovery, or even an amelioration of symptoms in this form of chorea; when once it begins it clings to the bitter end. No treatment seems to be of any avail, and indeed nowadays its end is so well known to the sufferer and his friends, that medical advice is seldom sought. It seems at least to be one of the incurables."

During his life, Huntington wrote just one paper, in rather old-fashioned style,[60] but it has remained a classic referred to by the renowned Canadian medical teacher William Osler in his textbook, the Principles and Practice of Medicine in 1893.[61]

One hundred and thirty years later the cause of Huntington's disease is still unknown. The diagnosis can be made both clinically and by genetic testing. The disease occurs world-wide and in about one in 20,000 persons. It continues from one generation to another, being inherited in an autosomal dominant manner, so that children have a 50 percent chance of developing "that disorder."[62,63] Genetic testing also allows presymptomatic detection of the disease but has profound social implications. In 1932, Vessie[64] showed that the disease in most patients in the eastern United States could be traced to six individuals who emigrated from the tiny village of Bures in Suffolk, England, 300 years earlier. Sadly, as Huntington wrote in 1872, "no treatment is of any avail."

11

ANTON CHEKHOV
(1860-1904)

Many people know that Anton Chekhov was a prolific writer of short stories and plays, but are unaware that he also practised as a doctor for most of his brief life of 44 years. His dual role widened his vision.

Born in 1860 at Taganrog near the Crimea, the third child of a strict father, he was naturally full of fun, but recalled, "There was no childhood in my childhood."[65] Indeed, when he woke every morning his first thought was, "Will I be beaten today?" During his early schooling he had to attend his father's grocery shop, endure the cold, wait on customers, take their money and replenish the supply of vodka for a favoured few...Meanwhile, Anton tried to complete his homework. There was no rest on Sunday, for the children had to attend church most of the day and sing in the choir.

Anton enjoyed his gentle mother's stories and developed a gift for story-telling himself, amusing his schoolmates. Attending a Greek church school he performed poorly at first, yet was stimulated by a

Father Pokrovksy[66] who loved literature and nurtured Anton's comic talent, encouraging him to read Molière, Swift and Russian satirist, Saltykov-Shchedrin.

At the age of 13 Anton discovered the theatre, delighting in make-believe and dressing-up, acting with his brothers in comic plays. Theatre provided an antidote for his home life. At sixteen, his life took a more serious turn when his father became bankrupt, sold their home and fled to Moscow to avoid a debtor's prison. Meanwhile Anton was left behind and had to live in his own home as a paying boarder. He finished high school, surviving by coaching students and even won a modest scholarship. Chekhov's background contrasted that of most Russian writers such as Turgenev, Pushkin and Tolstoy who emerged from a more secure environment.

Anton's first desire to study medicine probably followed a serious spell of peritonitis when he was fifteen, being influenced by his doctor's attentive care and his stories of medical student days.[67] Later his mother encouraged him to study medicine, writing from Moscow, "...apply to the Medical school. Medicine is the best career. Remember, Antosha, if you work hard you will always be able to earn a living in Moscow."[68]

In 1879 at the age of nineteen, Chekhov entered the Medical Faculty at Moscow University. It was an exciting time to be a medical student for medical teaching had been stimulated by the recent pathological and public health studies of Virchow which we noted in chapter eight, by the influence of Lister's antisepsis, (chapter three), and the advent of anesthesia. Professor Zakharin was professor of medicine. He emphasised detailed history-taking, the evolution of symptoms and the personal life, occupation, and psychological state of the patient.[69] Such an approach stimulated Chekhov who was already interested in the tales people told and the details of their lives. He became an industrious, quiet student. Meanwhile, he began to write amusing, snappy stories for the humour magazines to enable his family to survive. Arriving in Moscow he found them penniless, existing in one room in Moscow's "red light" district. At this stage Anton had no literary ambitions, he just wanted to make some easy money.[70]

However, it was not that easy to write perched on the edge of a chair while his family and friends bustled around him. His first pieces were rejected, but then <u>Dragon-fly</u> accepted one, and although they paid only five kopecks a line, he was on his way. Meanwhile he had to keep up with his medical studies.

Anton's father was frequently away so young Anton became the family's leader from whom all sought advice. Soon he was enabled by his writing and his scholarship to move the family into better lodgings. His writing conditions were still terrible, as he noted to Nikolai Leikin, editor of <u>Fragments</u> in August 1883.[71]

"I'm writing under abominable conditions. Before me sits my nonliterary work pummelling mercilessly away at my conscience, the fledgling of a visiting kinsman is screaming in the room next door.... Someone has wound up the music box, and I can hear La Belle Hélène... It makes me want to slip off to the country, but it's already one in the morning."

Nevertheless, he wrote. His earlier stories have not come down to us, but by 1883 he was scribbling out wonderful stories, humorous, satirical ones such as "<u>Death of a Civil Servant</u>", "<u>At the Post-Office</u>" and "<u>The Chameleon</u>"[72] and later some darker tales such as "<u>Misery,</u> "[73] sometimes called "<u>Heartache</u>." The <u>Chameleon</u> depicts a market square, empty of people while Police Inspector Moronoff and a constable stride across it. A dog squeals as a man, Grunkin, chases it and falling, grabs its leg. A crowd springs up from nowhere. "Looks like trouble, your honour!" says the constable. In the midst of the crowd, "sits the actual cause of the commotion: a white Borzoi puppy with a pointed muzzle and a yellow patch on its back. The expression in its watering eyes is one of terror and despair."[72]

Grunkin complains the dog bit his finger while he was walking along minding his own business. He wants time off from work and compensation. The Inspector wants to know who let the dog loose. He orders his constable to destroy it. Then an onlooker shouts it looks like General Tartaroff's dog, and the inspector quickly changes his tune, turns to Grunkin, "How would it reach up to your finger? a little dog like that... you skinned your finger on a nail, then had the bright idea of making some money out of it."

Onlookers argue back and forth. Apparently, Grunkin shoved

a cigarette in its face. The inspector wavers, but, fearing the General, releases the puppy to the General's cook and, warning Grunkin, "I'll deal with you later," strides off again across the square.

Meanwhile, Chekhov continued his medical studies. In 1879 he had pictured the University "as a sort of Greek temple basking in the sun of knowledge,"[74] and was amazed to discover a jumble of dark, dilapidated buildings. He found his fellow students long-haired and slovenly-looking. "We're just like school boys, regurgitating what we memorize and forgetting it as quickly as possible."[74]

Nevertheless, he was motivated to study hard, to attend the lectures and laboratories and to read widely. He avoided his fellow-students' political protests, believing that Russians should pull themselves up by their own bootstraps. Social progress should follow the will and education of the individual,[75] not mass hysteria.

Rossolimo, a fellow student and later professor of neuropathology at Moscow, recalled Chekhov's natural ease at obtaining a patient's case history including its intimate details.[76] During the summer Anton worked at a country hospital in Voskresensk under a Dr. Archangelesky who also noted how Anton listened quietly to his patients, never raising his voice however tired he was and even if the patient was talking about things seemingly "irrelevant to his illness.... The mental state of the patient interested him particularly."[77] For relaxation he went fishing. Also he hunted for usable characters in his stories at the post-office, tavern, peasants' quarters or gentry's mansions.[78]

In May 1884, Chekhov completed his exams and left for Voskresensk where his first fees came from treating a young woman with toothache, an actress with an unsettled stomach and a monk with dysentery.[77] Returning to Moscow he placed a copper plaque, "Anton Chekhov Medical Doctor" on his door and began to see mostly impecunious patients, students, artists and family friends. Working long hours that winter, he developed a dry cough and spasms of blood-spitting on December 7, 1884. He denied he had tuberculosis.[79]

Troyat noted that while writing, "Moving from story to story, he unconsciously painted a broad yet minute, humble yet faithful canvas of contemporary Russian life. There they were, side by side–the ordinary people he had caught unawares in both town and country: ignorant and brutal peasants, idle gentry folk half ruined by the emancipation of the serfs, drunken students with grand but naive ideas, disenchanted professors, unlucky doctors, shopkeepers chained to their accounts, corrupt officials. Society's loose change."[80]

For five years, Anton had treated his writing as a game to produce a necessary income and continued under a series of pseudonyms even after celebrated writer Nikolai Leskov had anointed him, "the way Samuel anointed David," during a drunken tour of Moscow night clubs in October 1883, and predicted a great future.[81] Nikolai Leikin, editor of Fragments, had urged Anton to write concisely and quickly. Now Leikin invited him to Petersburg and introduced him to Alexei Suvorin, editor of the influential journal New Times, to the venerable Dimitry Grigorovich and several others.

On March 25, 1886 Grigorovich wrote to Chekhov, gently chiding him for using a pseudonym and for not taking more time over his stories.[82] He informed Anton that he had outstanding talent and a great future if he learned to work slowly, carefully and conscientiously. "Stop trying to meet deadlines."

Chekhov replied hastily,[83]

"Your letter, my kind and dearly beloved bearer of glad tidings, struck me like a thunderbolt...May God comfort you in your old age as you have befriended my youth." He went on to explain that he was a doctor, "up to his ears in medicine," and could rarely write for more than two hours at a time.

In 1887, Anton experienced a spell of depression not alleviated by the success of a collection of his stories, At Twilight, for which he received the Pushkin prize for literature the following year. To help work his way out of his depression Anton started to compose a play, Ivanov, completing its first version within three weeks.

Not surprisingly, perhaps, the main character Ivanov, an exhausted and bored landowner, suffered from depression. He tells Dr. Lvov in Act I Scene III,

"Doctor, I'm so fed up with it all. I'm quite ill. I'm irritable, bad-tempered and rude these days, and so touchy, I hardly know myself. I have headaches for days on end, I can't sleep, and my ears buzz. But what can I do? Not a thing."[84]

Dr. John Coope, a North-of-England general practitioner who spent a lifetime researching Chekhov,[68] and even visited Russia with his wife, consulting original documents, pointed out in his intriguing 1997 biography that Chekhov at intervals throughout the play noted Ivanov's changing behaviour and significant pointers to a clinical picture which today is termed "endogenous depression," that is depression without an obvious external cause.

Chekhov's descriptions did not follow lectures that he had heard, but rather his own observations on people. In a long letter to his publisher, Suvorin, Anton defended the characters he created in the play. They "are the result of observing and studying life. They are still in my mind, and I feel I haven't lied a bit or exaggerated an iota."[85]

In the play, Ivanov's wife is dying of tuberculosis while Sasha, the young daughter of a neighbour falls in love with Ivanov and seeks to cure his moods. Ivanov, once energetic but now trapped in his depression, treats both women badly, and Dr. Lvov, the all-knowing recently graduated doctor lectures him. Ivanov considers his advice superficial.

"You think I am an open book, don't you.... Man's such a simple, uncomplicated mechanism. No, Doctor, we all have too many wheels, screws and valves to judge each other on first impressions or one or two pointers. I don't understand you, you don't understand me and we don't understand ourselves...." (Act III, scene VI.)[86]

After inadequate rehearsals, the actors did not understand their characters either, or even know their lines. Many drank between acts, behaving like clowns as the play progressed during opening night in Moscow. Naturally, the audience could not fathom the play. Hissing, clapping and arguments broke out among the audience before the play ended with Ivanov shooting himself. The police had to be called to restore order.[87]

Discouraged by its apparent failure and his powerlessness to influence its interpretation, Anton gave up play-writing for a while and returned to his tales and even to his childhood. Spending more time improving his stories, he finished just ten in 1888.[88] Among them was a longer tale, The Steppe. He informed Grigorovich,

"For my thick-journal I've selected the steppe, which no one has described for some time now. I describe the plain, its lilac vistas, the sheep breeders, the Jews, the priests, the nocturnal storms, the inns, the wagon trains, the steppe birds and so on ... There are passages that smell of hay...."[89]

Chekhov described the steppe through the wonder of shy nine-year-old Yegor, unconsciously no doubt using his childhood experiences slowly crossing the steppe by sturdy peasant wagon to visit his paternal grandfather, (incidentally named Yegor.) At night by the camp fire, "Watching the flames, Anton felt his heart overflow with gratitude for the clear sky above, the fragrance of grass and smoke, and his shivering kith and kin."[90]

The thick-journal was the Northern Herald. He worried that his Steppe's scenes "piled up on one another,"[89] but the editor accepted it with enthusiasm. Anton now felt written out. He just wanted to lie in bed and "spit on the ceiling," as the Russian saying goes.[91]

During the summers, Chekhov rented an estate for his family, socialised and wrote. Meanwhile, peasants who could not pay and others consulted him, so his life remained hectic. Returning to Moscow in September he started coughing blood again. "There is something ominous about blood coming from the mouth like the glow of a fire," he wrote to Suvorin,[92] and in another letter on September 11, 1888.[93] "You advise me not to chase after two hares at once and forget about practising medicine... but I feel more alert and more satisfied with myself as having two occupations rather than one... Medicine is my lawful wedded wife, and literature my mistress..."

He rewrote his Ivanov, which produced in Petersburg now proved a smashing success. He found the unexpected success, applause, a banquet in his honour and family responsibilities all exhausted him. He cared for his artist brother, Nikolai, now dying from typhus and tuberculosis. Watching him waste away he considered his own fate. His new play, The Wood Demon failed, and he was dissatisfied with himself.

Then, toward the end of 1889 he happened to pick up some notes on criminal law which his brother Mikhail had taken. Once the criminal is in prison, Anton thought, we forget about him. Suddenly he had a new aim. He would travel to the Russian penal colony on the island of

Sakhalin off the Eastern Siberian coast and do a scientific study on the convicts. Also, he hoped to submit it as a doctoral thesis. His family and friends were aghast. Could he survive the long hazardous journey across Russia?

But Chekhov, aided by his sister Maria's researches, had read about the millions of people "we have allowed to rot in jails." In a letter to Suvorin, March 1890, he commented, "We have let them rot to no purpose, unthinkingly and barbarously. We have driven people through the cold, in chains, across tens of thousands of versts, we have infected them with syphilis, debauched them, bred criminals and blamed it all on red-nosed prison wardens." And, "I want to write at least one or two hundred pages to pay off my debt to medicine, to which, as you know, I've behaved like a pig.[94]

There were other possible motives for his trip. He may have wanted to escape family responsibilities, his hectic Moscow social life with long nights of drinking with other writers in smoke-filled night clubs,[95] and perhaps Lydia Avilova who was in love with him.

In any event, he obtained initial permission from Galkin-Vrasky, head of the national prison administration, and, after extensive further study and preparations left for Sakhalin on April 21, 1890. He travelled first by train, then by boat, by tarantass, a sort of wicker basket harnessed to two horses, and finally a carriage. The tarantass hurt his back, for in icy conditions he was bumped along the ground for twelve days, but escaped more serious injury when his vehicle collided with three coaches coming in the opposite direction.[96] He forded floods, passed small groups of chained convicts, worn out from plodding along in their leg-irons, and eventually arrived at Lake Baikal with its transparent turquoise water, appreciating its views and those along the Amur river. Gold had been discovered. As usual Chekhov talked with all he met, noting in a letter to his sister Maria[97] that women smoked and people freely spoke their minds without fearing spies. He found minimal medical care available for the local population. By the roadside Anton examined a Jew with cancer of the liver. "He was exhausted and could hardly breathe, but that didn't stop the district nurses from applying 12 huge blood-sucking leeches."[98] He informed

Suvorin that he was keeping up with his medical practice.[99] One man asked him to examine his pregnant wife, and a mother her child.

Finally arriving at the coast on July 8th he viewed the island of Sakhalin across the water, "a fearful picture, crudely cast out of the darkness... monstrous bonfires, above them mountains, and from behind the mountains a crimson glow rising high in the sky...as if the whole of Sakhalin were ablaze...everything was covered in smoke as if we were in hell."[100]

Next day he crossed over to Alexandrovsk, the administrative capital and secured lodgings. Except for the clanking of chains among walking prisoners the streets were quiet.[101] Still, Chekhov was uncertain whether he would be allowed to talk with the prisoners.[100] Fortunately, the Governor received him courteously, and gave him permission to see all but political prisoners.

He impressed upon Chekhov the reasonable conditions in which the convicts lived and his personal aversion to corporal punishment. However, Chekhov soon found convicts chained to wheelbarrows working on their stomachs in the mines. "The Alexandrovsk hospital lacked the most elementary medicines, and patients slept on plank beds or on the floor. Prisoners were forbidden to enter churches. The guards reigned over their putrid charges with injustice, inhumanity and complete impunity....[102] Prisoners soon lost their sense of human dignity; they robbed one another, informed on one another."

As for the Governor's aversion to corporal punishment, Chekhov forced himself to attend a flogging in which the convict received 90 lashes, five at a time, the flogger moving slowly from side to side to side, striking the victim diagonally, peeling the skin with each blow.

"Suddenly his neck stretched out unnaturally, and we heard vomiting...He did not say another word; he only moaned and wheezed." Chekhov could stand it no longer, escaping into the street. But, the screams followed him and the horror reappeared to him in dreams. [102] He found it hard to believe that the Governor was unaware of these floggings.

To perform his census among the prisoners, Chekhov had small cards printed in the Police Department,[103] and, working from dawn to dusk, usually accompanied by an armed guard, he managed to question some 10,000 inhabitants, filling in their answers to 13 basic questions, including name, marriage status, relation to head of household, birth date, if a child, whether legitimate or not, literacy, etc. The year of their arrival was such a terrible misfortune to prisoners that many could not remember it.[103]

While talking with individuals, the general gloom was occasionally lightened. "Why are your dog and cockerel tied up?" I would ask a householder.

"Here on Sakhalin everything's chained up," he'd crack a reply. "It's that sort of place."[104]

Chekhov found fairly similar conditions throughout the region, although in Dué and Voyevodsk men were dreadfully overcrowded and shackled to iron balls.[105]

Some wives had accompanied their husbands to Sakhalin voluntarily. Many women were forced to practise prostitution in order to survive. Most of the island's children were emaciated and illiterate. If convicts survived their prison term they had to remain in the colony. They were not allowed back into Russia. Convicts made numerous escape attempts although well aware of the harsh treatment on recapture. Tuberculosis, syphilis and other diseases were common.

By October 13, 1890 Chekhov had completed his census and while proud of his accomplishment was relieved to leave convicts, chains and misery, and return home which he did by sea via Hong Kong and Ceylon. Writing his detailed factual report bored him, and more than once he was tempted to abandon it. Furthermore, he had used up his borrowed funds during the trip and needed to write for profit.

Meanwhile, a famine was developing in the Russian countryside. A world-wide agricultural crisis, savage Government fiscal policies and inefficient land use all contributed. By the autumn of 1891, many peasants were eating "famine bread" composed of rye and goose foot, a weed without nutritional value which caused diarrhoea and further protein loss.[106]

Chekhov "hurled himself frantically into relief work for the outlying provinces,"[107] thereby reducing his time for writing. Then cholera broke out in the summer of 1892 and the local district council asked Chekhov to take charge of efforts to prevent its spread.[108] He had isolation barracks built, sought funds from neighbours or rich factory owners and jolted from village to village teaching suspicious peasants about the disease, meanwhile treating patients with typhus, diphtheria and scarlet fever. The sick were still his primary concern.

Chekhov's regimen for the active treatment of cholera included replacing fluids by warm tannin enemas and subcutaneous injections of table salt.[109] Fortunately, the epidemic did not reach Melikhovo, where he had purchased an estate in February, 1892, partly to live more economically. While at Melikhovo he wrote some twenty-seven stories including Peasants[110] in which he described the sordid realities of peasant life and their need for poverty relief. On publication it caused an uproar. Another story, Ward number six, was a gloomy tale about a provincial mental hospital doctor who loses his initial enthusiasm and eventually becomes a patient brutalised by the powerful warder.

He continued to labour on his Sakhalin study. Finally in 1893, after censorship by the Central Prison Department, the first three chapters were serialised in Russian Thought and later chapters excepting 21 and 22, forbidden by the censor, followed through 1894. Chekhov was careful to write objectively. The final version was published in 1895.[111]

Karlinsky commented[112] that The Island of Sakhalin was favourably reviewed by the Russian press. "A wealth of documentation proves that Chekhov's book was instrumental in bringing about much-needed reforms in the penal-colony administration and that it helped improve the conditions under which the convict-settlers lived." However, when Chekhov's friend Grigory Rossolimo, Professor of Neuropathology at Moscow asked the dean of the medical school whether the study could be accepted for his doctorate in medicine, the dean... "turned around and walked out without saying a word."[112] In 1896, Chekhov completed another play, The Seagull in which a group of people including two writers, two actresses and a doctor gather at an estate by the lakeshore. Their fantasies fail against the rocks of everyday existence.[113] The writer Trigorin replies to the beautiful actress, Nina, in Act 11, possibly portraying Chekhov's own experiences.

"Yes, writing's pleasant enough...but as soon as the stuff's in print I can't stand it – I now see it was all wrong, all a mistake, and shouldn't have been written at all...The public reads it and says, 'Yes. Oh, how nice. Oh, how clever... but not a patch on Tolstoy.'"[113]

On its opening night, the audience, looking forward to the next play, a three-act-comedy, failed to appreciate Chekhov's psychological nuances and booed. Chekhov fled the theatre and wandered through the dark streets.

In March the following year, continuing his medical workload Anton experienced a huge hemorrhage and needed to enter a pulmonary clinic under Dr. Alexei Ostroumov who insisted he stop practising medicine and live a quieter life. Next year, 1898, after a period of rest he defied medical orders and busied himself writing and seeing patients again at Melikhovo. But, by the end of summer he lost his energy and returned to Moscow where he attended theatre rehearsals and became impressed by the beauty and talent of a young actress, Olga Knipper. However, more spells of coughing forced him to convalesce in the south at Yalta.

One is tempted to write much more on Chekhov, of his courting Olga and their eventual marriage; of his selfless sister, Maria; of his friendship with writers Maxim Gorky and the immortal Tolstoy; of his later stories such as The Lady with the Dog, In the Ravine and The Betrothed; and of his recently discovered stories;[114] of his link with the Moscow Art Theatre and his final three plays. Uncle Vanya, (1899,) The Three Sisters, (1901) and the Cherry Orchard, (1904.) Slowly audiences began to appreciate his unorthodox plays and their inner meaning. His final play concerned the decline of an estate and a passing of the old ways. He completed it by sheer will-power, a few lines at a time between spells of breathlessness and coughing blood.

But it would take too much space to describe the material thoroughly. I would rather conclude with his stated writing principles and with his words from two earlier tales.

To his friend and classmate Grigory Rossolimo he declared in 1899,[115] "...my study of medicine has had a serious impact on my literary activities. It significantly broadened the scope of my observations and enriched me with knowledge whose value for me as a writer only a doctor can appreciate. It also served as a guiding influence... My familiarity with the natural sciences and the scientific method has always kept me on my guard...."

In his stories, Chekhov avoided preaching. He let his characters speak for themselves and left his readers to draw their own conclusions. Eleven years earlier he commented to Alexei Pleshcheyev,[116] "I am neither liberal, nor conservative...I would like to be a free artist...My holy of holies is the human body, health, intelligence, talent, inspiration, love and the most absolute freedom imaginable, freedom from violence and lies, no matter what form the latter two take."

Two stories illustrate Chekhov's sensitive understanding of the human psyche. In <u>Misery</u> (1886) an old sleigh driver Iona, sits waiting for a fare, "bent as double as a living body can be bent," while flakes of soft wet snow cover him and his mare white.[73] At last three boisterous young men hire him. "Get on, you old plague," they order him. Eventually there is a pause in their conversation and the old man, who has been longing to speak, says, "This week... er ... my ... er ... son died!" His fares show not the slightest interest. "We shall all die,..." comments one. "Come, drive on! Drive on!"

Later his passengers leave. Again he is alone. The misery which was eased a little by their presence now "tears his heart more cruelly than ever..." Among the crowds can he not find "someone who will listen to him? But the crowds flit by..." Later he tries to talk to a cabman in the yard, but his words have no effect.

Finally he feeds his mare and talks to her. "That's how it is, old girl... He went and died for no reason... now, suppose you had a little colt, and you were a mother to that little colt... And all at once that same little colt went and died... You'd be sorry wouldn't you?...."

"The little mare munches, listens, and breathes on her master's hands. Iona is carried away and tells her everything."

A <u>Doctor's Visit</u> (1898,) also reveals the healing power of narrative.[117] Liza, a 20-year-old factory owner and only daughter of Madame Lyalikov is ill. The Moscow professor, too busy to consult, sends his assistant, Korolyov who is charmed by the drive from the station but appalled by the ugliness of the worker's environment, "all covered with a film of grey dust."

The distraught elderly mother, governess and Korolyov enter the invalid's room. "I have heart palpitations," she says. "It was so awful last night....I almost died of fright! Do give me something."

He examines and reassures her. Suddenly, Liza puts her hands to her head and, along with her mother, burst into sobs. Korolyov no longer notices her ugliness. She now seems "graceful and feminine." He longs to soothe her, "not with drugs or advice but with simple kindly words."

They beg him to stay the night. Later, walking outside, he considers the depressing factories, the workers, their working conditions, wretched cheap cotton goods and the owner's unhappiness. In the stillness of the night, the watchman striking the hour by an unpleasant clanking on a sheet of metal seems like "the Devil himself, who controlled the owners and the workers alike, and was deceiving both."

Returning to the house he finds Liza still awake. They talk. "Everything worries me... it seemed to me as soon as I saw you I knew I could tell you about it." She wanted to talk, not with a doctor, but with some intimate friend who would understand her... "I am so lonely...."

Now it was clear to him that she should give up her factories and her profits. But how to say it? They discuss the problem in a roundabout way, but she has the opportunity to reveal her inner tale.

Next morning the family sees him off. Liza wears a white dress and a flower in her hair. The doctor thinks, "how pleasant it was on such a morning in the spring to drive with three horses in a good carriage, and bask in the sunshine."

In his quiet ending Chekhov uses the woman's coverings to reveal the healing potential of narrative.

12

WILLIAM CARLOS WILLIAMS (1883-1963)

William Carlos Williams could not make up his mind. Born and raised in Rutherford, New Jersey, he had entered the University of Pennsylvania to study medicine in 1902, after two earlier years in Europe and finishing high school at Horace Mann in New York. However, no sooner had he begun his medical studies, he wanted to quit them and devote himself to writing.[118]

It was at Horace Mann that Williams first studied poetry. His teacher, William Abbott, fondly known as Uncle Billy, inspired him with poetry and "the excitement of great books."[119] Also, during his first year Williams tried out for track, but, sprinting one turn too early during practice, collapsed at the finish line. His family doctor advised that he had strained his heart and forbade further competition. Williams, who had hoped to be a track star at the school, fell into a depression. His first poem then "came" to him, a poem which both described his mood and gave him mysterious joy.

A black, black cloud
flew over the sun
driven by fierce flying
rain.

The joy he felt was partly mitigated by his critical analysis. How could clouds be driven by rain? Stupid.[120]

His younger brother Ed, to whom he remained close, was studying architecture at the Massachusetts Institute of Technology. He had an English Professor named Arlo Bates with whom he discussed his "literary brother." An appointment was arranged.

Williams arrived with a long rolled-up poem, composed after the style of Keats. Fumbling, he dropped it on the floor before the great man; Williams anxiously awaited his opinion.

"You have a sensitive appreciation of the work of John Keat's line and form," Bates commented, then advised him to go on with his medical studies. Pulling out a drawer in his desk, he continued, "I, too, write poems. And when I have written them I place them here–and– then I close the drawer."[118]

Williams thanked him and left with his mind more settled. Medicine would provide the necessary income to let him write unfettered.

At the University he formed friendships with, among others, the gifted and erratic writer Ezra Pound, Hilda Doolittle and painter Charles Demuth. He intended to specialize and completed two and a half years of hectic internship in New York, emphasising general medicine, obstetrics, (when he delivered over 300 babies), and pediatrics. His spell at the Nursery and Child's hospital at Sixty-first Street and Tenth Avenue was cut short when he refused to sign a report after not being allowed to see the original figures of a hospital business matter. Graft had occurred. The other doctors had always signed them, he was told. But, that was not good enough for Williams who happened at the same time to be ill with a sore throat and high fever. His principles cost him a specialty career in New York.[121]

However, working-class immigrants around Paterson and Rutherford where he later started practice became the beneficiaries of his thorough training. Meanwhile, he proposed to his future wife,

Flossie Herman, and then spent the next year exploring Europe, the arts and medicine.

His years in Europe and his parents, English father and French-Dutch–Spanish–Jewish mother from Martinique, encouraged his wider vision. Later he noted that men gave him the direction of his life, while women supplied the energy.[118]

Like Chekhov, his medical observations strongly influenced his writing. No doubt it was after visiting a patient at home that he compiled his simple, yet profound poem, "The Red Wheel-barrow."[122]

So much depends
upon
a red wheel
barrow
glazed with rain water
beside the white
chickens.

Williams made a habit of writing down a phrase which might come to him at any time.

"I was permitted by my medical badge to follow the poor, defeated body into those gulfs and grottoes. And the astonishing thing is that at such times and in such places–foul as they may be with the stinking ischio-rectal abscesses of our comings and goings–, just there, the thing, in all its greatest beauty, may for a moment be freed to fly for a moment guiltily about the room. In illness, in the permission I as a physician have had to be present at deaths and births, at the tormented battles between daughter and diabolic mother, shattered by a gone brain–just there–for a split second–from one side or the other, it has fluttered before me for a moment, a phrase which I quickly write down on anything at hand, any piece of paper I can grab."[123] Later the poem would flow from the phrase or phrases. He would bang the poem out on his typewriter between patients or when he was tired, coming home after a night call. Often when he was tired from medical work he wrote freely. He wrote sensitively from direct experience.

Early in his writing, he decided to begin his poems with lower-case letters and not to rhyme. His poems therefore looked different and sounded different; they were of ordinary things viewed with empathy and honesty, and were intended to interest ordinary readers, contrasting for example the intellectual poetry of Eliot in "The Waste Land" with its pages of footnotes,[124] returning the poem to the academics.

For example, Williams noted a "Poor Old Woman"[125]

munching a plum on
the street a paper bag
of them in her hand

they taste good to her
they taste good
to her. They taste
good to her
You can see it by
the way she gives herself
to the one half
sucked out in her hand

Comforted
a solace of ripe plums
seeming to fill the air
They taste good to her

He noticed a rumpled sheet of brown paper rolling with the wind, and described it in "The Term."[126]

...
a car drove down
upon it and
crushed it to
the ground. Unlike
a man it rose
again rolling
with the wind over
and over to be as
it was before.

He concluded his poem, "The Rose"[127]

...

The fragility of the flower
unbruised
penetrates space.

He was close to his grandmother, and his poem about "The Last Words of My English Grandmother," described her ending.[128]

....

Oh, oh, oh! she cried
as the ambulance men lifted
her to the stretcher–
Is this what you call
making me comfortable?
By now her mind was clear–
Oh you think you're smart
You young people,
she said, but I'll tell you
you don't know anything.
Then we started
on the way

We passed a long row
of elms. She looked at them
a while out of
the ambulance window and said,
What are all those
fuzzy-looking things out there?
Trees? Well I'm tired
of them and rolled her head away.

William's verse, flavoured with an earthy sympathetic social realism, contributed a distinctive nonacademic element to American poetry and exerted a huge influence upon developing avant garde poetry. However, most critics disliked it. As Randall Jarell observed in 1949, "Contemporary criticism has not done very well by Williams; most of the good critics of poetry have not written about him, and one or two of the best, when they did write, just twitched as if flies were crawling over them."[129]

Williams ignored the critics and continued writing. Meanwhile he laboured at his medical practice. At one time during those years he "gave birth" as one woman phrased it, to nearly every baby born on those streets above the old copper mines.[130] It was a rough neighbourhood. After one home birth at three in the morning, the husband suggested he ride back with Williams. Later Williams noted the gun in his pocket. The man explained that he had seen a couple of his wife's cousins looking at Williams's car. "They are no good. But, if they knew I was with you they wouldn't bother you," he added.

On another occasion Williams was called to a difficult delivery by another doctor, exhausted after a 24 hour labour in a huge woman. Williams was met at the door by her irate husband who soon brandished a "45" and threatened to shoot both doctors if either his wife or baby were harmed. Fortunately, Williams had kept up with medical advances and had brought with him a new drug, pituitrin. The woman's contractions had ceased, but minutes after one shot of pituitrin, amidst cries and curses she expelled two large babies into a hostile world.[131]

Williams continued his regular post-graduate work, attending mostly pediatric clinics in New York, and sometimes spending the evening afterwards with poet and painter friends. Their poems were constantly rejected by the regular paying magazines, so they started their own "little magazines" which lasted for short periods.

Flossie and he had two children and proved sociable hosts for many years at 9 Ridge Road in Rutherford, New Jersey. The family survived the 1918 "flu," and in 1924 took a year's sabbatical, partly in Europe, spending much of the time with relatives or artist friends.[132] During the year he wrote In the American Grain, consisting of a series of lively historical vignettes of people entering the Americas. He showed great sympathy for the original inhabitants. "History! History! We fools, what do we know or care? History begins for us with murder or enslavement, not with discovery." The book sold poorly. Later, during the depression years when his practice dwindled, he had more time for writing and finished The White Mule,[133] a story of immigrants based partly on the Hermans, his wife's family. The novel was well-reviewed and the first edition quickly sold. Unfortunately, his publisher, James Laughlin, was away in New Zealand, skiing for the US team, so timely production of more copies was delayed.

Many readers would enjoy Williams's short stories. When describing his medical experiences he often reached a white hot intensity, as for example in The Use of Force.[134]

Called to see a new patient's only daughter, Williams tried to examine her on her father's lap in the kitchen. "I could see that they were all very nervous eying me up and down distrustfully. As often in such cases, they weren't telling me more than they had to, it was up to me to tell them; that's why they were spending three dollars on me."

"The child was fairly eating me up with her cold, steady eyes..."

"'She's had a fever for three days,' began the father, 'and we don't know what it comes from.... So we tho't you'd better look her over and tell us what is the matter'."

"As doctors often do I took a trial shot at it as a point of departure. 'Has she had a sore throat?'"

"Both parents answered me together, 'No... No, she says her throat don't hurt her.'"

"'Does your throat hurt you?' added the mother to the child. But the little girl's expression didn't change nor did she move her eyes from my face."

"'Have you looked?'"

"I tried to, said the mother, but I couldn't see."

"There had been a number of cases of diphtheria at her school. And we were all, quite apparently thinking of that, though no one had as yet spoken of the thing,"

They tried to coax the girl to open her mouth. Nothing doing.

....Slowly I approached the child again. As I moved my chair a little nearer suddenly with one cat-like movement both her hands clawed instinctively for my eyes and she almost reached them too. In fact she knocked my glasses flying. The parents were abject in their apology and angry with their daughter. "'You bad girl...look what you've done. The nice man....'"

"For heaven's sake I broke in. Don't call me a nice man to her. I'm here to look at her throat on the chance she might have diphtheria and possibly die of it. But that's nothing to her....'"

"I had to have a throat culture for her own protection." Williams continued, "I had already fallen in love with the savage brat....'"

The father tried his best to hold her still but released her too early just at the critical point. Williams fought to push a wooden tongue depressor between her teeth. She reduced it to splinters. Her tongue and mouth were cut. She screamed in hysterical shrieks. "But I must get a diagnosis... ...the worst of it was that I too had got beyond reason. I could have torn the child apart in my own fury and enjoyed it... The damned little brat must be protected against her own idiocy."

Eventually, Williams overpowered her jaws with his hands and a heavy silver spoon, and saw both tonsils covered with a diphtheritic membrane. He had discovered her secret. Now she was furious and tried to attack the doctor again "while tears of defeat blinded her eyes."

Another remarkable tale was that of old Doc Rivers,[135] a doctor in the area who continued practising medicine and surgery and had a devoted following, in spite of his long addiction to morphine, heroin, and cocaine, and his periodic absences.

A Harvard doctor, Robert Coles, compiled some of these tales.[136] While a student he contacted Dr. Williams, and was invited to accompany him on his rounds. He became entranced by "Doc" Williams, by his tales, by his patients and by his caring honesty.[137] Later he used Williams' experiences and tales to give Harvard medical students a realistic view of medical practice.[135]

Recognition came late to Williams.[129] Over 30 years elapsed before some universities began to ask him to read his poetry. Fiercely loyal to America, he spoke at City College, New York, in 1943 of Americans' right to define their own language. An instructor, "an obvious Britisher," questioned the origins of Americans' language. "Where does it come from?" he asked.

"From the mouths of Polish mothers," Williams countered.[138]

Williams believed it imperative "that the American poet not

follow the classic forms but invent his own."[139] In that way only would Americans ever have a chance of creating work comparable to the classics. Recognition of his medical talents came later still, following Robert Coles's visits to Williams in the early fifties, after Williams had practised steadily for over 40 years and after his first stroke.[137] As Coles observed,[140] "Words were the instrument of grace given to this one doctor, and words are the instrument of grace, also, for the rest of us, the readers who have and will come upon these marvelously provocative tales."

In his long prose-poem Paterson,[141] over which he laboured many years, Williams described the life of the city and its people from the start of the century into the fifties. The immigrants, poverty, assembly lines, industrial strife, the nearby river, park, sexuality, politics, a murder, his patients–his teachers. Pride, arrogance, greed, hypocrisy, courage, love. All life. For Williams poetry and medicine were nearly the same thing.[142]

He was awarded the Pulitzer prize posthumously for his poetic work, Pictures from Brueghel. He had produced some 50 works of poetry and prose. At the end he was weak and unable to read. Flossie continued to care for him and read to him hour after hour though her vocal cords were raw. After he died she wrote to their friend Marianne Moore that she and Bill had had a good life together - in fact a life.[143] His son Eric took over his practice.

Williams never worried that medicine interfered with his work as a writer. "Was I not interested in man? There the thing was, right in front of me. I could touch it, smell it. It was myself, naked...."[143]

"What is the use of reading the common news of the day, the tragic deaths and abuses of daily living... It is a trivial stop-gap... But the haunted news I get from some obscure patient's eyes is not trivial....

"It is just a glimpse, an intimation of all that which the daily print misses or deliberately hides.... It is then we see, by this constant feeling for a meaning, from the unselected nature of the material, just as it comes in over the phone or at the office door, that there is no better way to get an intimation of what is going on in the world."[144]

"My business, aside from the mere physical diagnosis is to make a different sort of diagnosis concerning them as individuals... That fascinates me."

"Do we not see that we are inarticulate? That is what defeats us. It is our inability to communicate to another how we are locked within ourselves, unable to say the simplest thing of importance to one another."

His phrase reminds us of another general practitioner, Chekhov, in his play Ivanov.[86]

"... I don't understand you, you don't understand me and we don't understand ourselves."

Robert Coles wrote of Williams, "He gives us permission to bare our souls, to be candidly introspective, but not least to smile at ourselves, to be grateful for the continuing opportunity we have to make recompense for our failures of omission or commission." [145]

Williams noted that,

"The relationship between physician and patient, if it were literally followed, would give us a world of extraordinary fertility of the imagination which we can hardly afford."

Like Chekhov, Williams well understood the meaning of "family medicine," "psychosomatic medicine," and "behavioural science," long before the terms became popular.[144,145] He was acutely aware of the effects of culture, mind, class, sexuality, values and environment upon health. He summarised his medical work in the chapter "The Practice,"[144]

"It's the humdrum, day-in, day-out, everyday work that is the real satisfaction of the practice of medicine... I have never had a money practice.... But the actual calling on people, at all times and under all conditions, the coming to grips with the intimate conditions of their lives, when they were being born, when they were dying, watching them die, watching them get well when they were ill, has always absorbed me. I lost myself in the very properties of their minds...."

If we truly wish to improve the quality of health care today, we could well start by studying William Carlos Williams.

I wish, while a student, I had been introduced to the work of Jenner, Chekhov and "Doc" Williams.

13

WILLIAM PICKLES
(1885-1969)

While considering the work of Chekhov and Williams we saw the close connection between mind and body in disease. Now let us return to essentially physical illness and particularly the common infectious diseases seen by general practitioners in their younger patients.

In 1913, William Pickles joined a practice in the village of Aysgarth in the Wensleydale district of Yorkshire, England. He became particularly interested in infectious illnesses after noting a gypsy woman start a local epidemic of typhoid fever by washing her sick husband's clothes at a faulty village pump.[146] Pickles cured the epidemic by having the village pump put out of action. In those days, current textbooks poorly described the incubation period and the natural history of many common childhood diseases such as measles, chicken-pox, mumps and scarlet fever. Pickles began to keep careful charts of his patients, noting the course of their illnesses and how they spread to other folk in the district. He began researching at the rather late age of 42, gradually recognising the advantages a country practitioner possessed, having a stable population to investigate and knowing nearly everyone in the village and something of their intimate relationships and their comings and goings.

In his lively little book, Epidemiology in Country Practice,[146] Pickles described how one summer evening he climbed to the top of a local hill and watched a train creep slowly up the valley, pausing at three stations.

"In the north-east, Mary Stuart's early prison, Bolton Castle, was lighted up by the setting sun, the attractive little lake, Semmerwater, appeared to lie at my feet, and one by one I made out most of our grey villages, with their thin cloud of smoke. In all those villages there was hardly a soul, man, woman, or child, of whom I did not, and do not, know even the Christian name, and every country doctor of long standing could say the same of his own district."

"This wide personal knowledge and love of the country in which we live fit even the most commonplace of us for epidemiological research, and I have known several country practitioners with useful knowledge to impart, gathered from their own observations, but who considered it too trivial even to write down, much less to publish. Nothing, I believe, is further from the truth, and by withholding these observations from the public, these men are damming up sources of information that are among the only accurate ones from which such information can be drawn."

One less common but important epidemic illness existed under different names in different localities,– "devil's grip," "epidemic myalgia," and "Bornholm disease." The illness often presented with severe abdominal pain or chest pain and thus could be mistaken for such diseases as acute appendicitis, intussusception or pneumonia.

Pickles and his partner first encountered the condition in July 1933. The concerned young father of a 2 1/2 year-old boy woke Pickles to ask him to see his son suffering from alarming upper abdominal pain. The boy was sweating, breathing rapidly and shallowly, and looked ill. He did not vomit or have diarrhoea or any skin rash. Later that day Pickles returned with his partner, Dr. Dunbar, to re-examine the child. His temperature had now risen to 101 F and he was breathing 60 times a minute. The doctors were not sure of the diagnosis but suspected early pneumonia.

However, next morning "the little rascal, standing on the window-sill and thumping on the window, greeted me smilingly, but I thought derisively, as I walked up the garden path."[147]

Pickles, to his surprise, now could find nothing wrong with the child. He admitted his ignorance to the mother but assured her not to worry any more about him.

"This was an extremely rash remark, as I was to learn to my cost later," he commented. Next morning the child appeared to be seriously ill again. Fortunately, by the evening of the next day, he recovered.

Meanwhile, two little girls who were constant companions of this boy and his two brothers, had visited him. Four days later, they too came down with similar symptoms. Furthermore, his two brothers had developed the illness. Four days after the children had recovered their father noticed a pain in his shoulder which soon increased in severity and spread to his rib margin and to his arms. He also experienced difficulty breathing. Examination disclosed tenderness over his lower ribs and upper abdominal muscles. His chest was clear.

Later Pickles discovered that a young visitor to the little girl's farm earlier had suffered severe spasm–like pains during her visit and had to lie down for the day. She seems to have been the original source of the infection.

The characteristics of the illness were its sudden onset and its episodic quality. A child would be quite well and be running about, then suddenly would collapse with pain, then seem to recover, then relapse. The illness lasted three or four days in each case.

The infectious nature of the illness and consistency of the tale told by the affected children along with the observations of their parents and physicians were confirmed by a Danish practitioner, Dr. Sylvest, with whom Pickles had corresponded the previous year about catarrhal jaundice. The new illness was quite common on the Danish island of Bornholm and Sylvest sent Pickles articles he had written about it. Sylvest had termed the disorder, "myositis epidemica" or "Bornholm disease."[148] The importance in recognising the disease lay in its similarity to more serious conditions. For example, Crone and

Chapman[149] recorded an epidemic of 30 cases at the Massachussets General Hospital in 1933 when two young patients were mistakenly operated upon for acute appendicitis and one other patient for a suspected perforated duodenal ulcer.[149]

Pickles studied the epidemiology of many other infectious diseases, including influenza, measles, sonne dysentery, scarlet fever, mumps, catarrhal jaundice, chicken-pox, herpes zoster and the relationship between the latter two diseases.

His wife and daughter helped with his case records and charts, while school teachers and his patients helped point out the possible spread of disease between patients thereby all becoming valuable research partners. Pickles himself studied the geology and water supply of the district and noted the history of past epidemics in the parish register.

After many rejections, John Wright of Bristol accepted his manuscript and published it in 1939. Sadly, many copies and the type were burned during an air raid on Bristol in 1941.[150] Fortunately, the Devonshire Press republished it later.

As for recent understanding of Bornholm disease, Harrison's textbook, 1998 edition, provides a brief, but similar clinical picture to Pickles, sixty years later. Most cases are caused by the coxsackievirus B, occur in epidemics, and resolve within four days.[151] The disease is still important to consider before operating on a possible intra-abdominal problem such as appendicitis. Pickles' modestly written work[146] continues to deserve close study. Pickles was influenced by another great general practitioner, James Mackenzie.

14

JAMES MACKENZIE
(1853-1925)

While encountering these tales I became impressed by the number of general practitioner researchers from the time of Jenner to the present. I have tried to describe the work of some well known practitioners and some less well known ones, from the UK and Europe and from the United States and Canada. I record only a sample of their work.

For example, a century after Jenner, Robert Koch (1843-1910),[152,153] a country doctor in Wollstein, Germany was disturbed by a disease that greatly affected his farming families and their flocks. Determined to find its cause he used a microscope behind a screen in his examining room to discover the anthrax bacillus, becoming in 1873 the first physician to show that a specific organism, the anthrax bacillus, caused a specific disease, anthrax. He identified both bacillus and its spores, grew it on artificial media such as agar and gelatin, and transmitted it through generations of mice. Recently, anthrax became a contemporary problem following the events of September 11th, 2001.

Koch also studied surgical wound infections and later in 1882, while working for the Imperial Health Department, discovered the tubercle bacillus, the cause of that dreaded scourge, tuberculosis.

In the UK, William Withering in 1785,[154,155] and James Mackenzie a century later, contributed significantly to our understanding of heart disease. Withering, an outstanding botanist as well as a physician, while listening to his patients paid attention to folk remedies, (as Jenner had done before him, chapter 9.) In 1775, he learned of a remedy for "the dropsy," (grossly swollen legs from fluid retention,) kept secret by an old Shropshire woman.[156] That remedy contained some twenty herbs, but Withering soon found the active ingredient to be digitalis, present in the common purple foxglove leaf. Later, he learned of its independent use in Warwickshire and in the western part of Yorkshire where people used to "cure themselves of dropsical complaints by drinking foxglove tea."[156]

Withering began using digitalis in dropsical cases in 1775. Well aware of its side-effects in too high dosage, namely vomiting, diarrhoea, visual changes and slowed pulse, he learned how to obtain a consistent dose of digitalis from the foxglove leaf. He carefully described his cases, including those where digitalis failed to help. Today, digitalis remains a valued remedy in some cases of "dropsy" and in some cases of heart disease.

James Mackenzie was born in Scone, Scotland in 1853. He was fortunate in his Presbyterian parents who stressed love and discipline. However, at school he found himself considered a "dunce" for failing to memorize.[157] Leaving school at 15 he first apprenticed to a pharmacist, working long hours.

Soon he found the work wearisome, but in later years considered it taught him endurance. Trudging home in the dark up a hill to his family's farm he would see in the distance the light of a lamp placed in the gable window by his mother to welcome him. He spent much of his little spare time reading. During his duties he would meet many doctors and those contacts may have stimulated him to become a doctor.

Entering Edinburgh medical school at the age of 22, he encountered again his old enemy – memorization. He enjoyed the later clinical years more for they included thought and problem solving. Later he wrote of his education,[158]

"In my career through college I always had the greatest difficulty keeping pace with the lecturers and seldom succeeded. Evidently, the standard, if there is a standard, which guides a teacher, is to pour out facts at a rate a little beyond the capacity of the student who has the most retentive memory... no student is able to absorb the whole knowledge, and most of them only a very small part of the knowledge.... I felt a longing to devote myself to some of the branches of medicine concerned in research, but my very moderate attainments precluded me from obtaining any of the coveted posts about the University, and I quite clearly recognised that I was only suited for what is considered the lowest place in the medical profession."

After graduating, he first worked as a locum in two practices, then spent six months as House physician to Professor Sanders at Edinburgh, and finally was welcomed by Dr. Brown and Dr. Briggs to their practice in Burnley, Lancashire during 1879. It proved a fortunate association.

Mackenzie soon found that his medical school teaching had oversimplified diseases as being easily identified by their symptoms and signs. He did not find his patients' problems so neatly categorised. Later, he observed,[159]

"The great majority of students of medicine become general practitioners, and in the teaching schools, with rare exceptions, there is not one teacher who has obtained a knowledge of many of the problems which will meet the general practitioner. Probably in this respect medical education is unique in that in all other branches of knowledge, whether a trade or profession, the teachers or instructors have a practical acquaintance with the subjects they teach...."

Although he studied all he could and sought his senior colleagues' welcome advice, he realised the answers he sought often did not exist. About 1882 he determined to find the answers and started by keeping careful notes on his patients.

He concentrated upon two problems, pain and irregular heart beat. Many patients suffered abdominal, particularly stomach ulcer pain. He asked one patient to clearly define where he felt the pain, then asked him to take a deep breath and indicate where the pain now was. During a deep breath the stomach's position moves, but the patient indicated that the position of his pain, (in the upper abdomen, - the epigastrium,) had not changed.[160] The skin in this area was tender. Clearly, the pain came from the skin and its sensory nerves not from the stomach.

Dr. James Ross of Manchester, whose work Mackenzie appreciated, believed that pain from a diseased organ came from that organ itself and not from the skin. But, operating upon another patient who refused any anesthetic, Mackenzie found that the patient experienced pain when his skin was cut, but no pain when a portion of his bowel was cut out or sutured. He did however experience pain while a normal peristaltic wave passed along the intestine. That pain he felt not where the bowel was - now lying to one side of the patient, but at the umbilicus, the centre of the abdomen.[161] Clearly, the pain was not coming from the organ itself.

Mackenzie mapped specific areas of the skin which became sensitive when underlying organs were diseased, such as tenderness in the right side of the upper abdomen, which he found in a patient with a stone in the bile duct, experiencing the pain of biliary colic. In 1882, he was awarded an M.D. for his thesis on a patient presenting with pain and numbness in his legs caused by syphilis of the spinal cord. He studied cases of herpes zoster (shingles) prior to the work of Henry Head who researched the same condition later, ignoring Mackenzie's earlier contributions.[162]

Mackenzie showed how the lesions and hypersensitivity in herpes zoster followed the distribution of the cutaneous nerves. He also noted that the areas of skin hypersensitivity were not as clearly demarcated as Head later described.

Years afterward, Professor Fraser Roberts of Guy's hospital in London heard the aging Mackenzie recall visiting a Burnley patient with shingles. During the visit he marked the reddened areas of skin with a pencil, and then after waiting awhile, found that some areas "previously red were now blanched and vice versa." He said, "I knew at that moment that Head and Rivers were wrong."[163]

Mackenzie's opinions developed from examining actual cases

in his practice. Nevertheless, the profession accepted Head's work on sensation and neglected Mackenzie. Eventually, Mackenzie's sheer volume of described patients with heart disease forced the profession to recognise the work of the Burnley general practitioner.

Mackenzie's life encompassed more than work. He entered into Burnley's social life, joining the Burnley Literary and Scientific Society and also played bridge, chess, billiards, tennis and later golf. In 1887 he met Frances Jackson, governess to four children, while making a home visit to one of the girls when she was ill. Frances was impressed by his genuine affection for his little patient. Later, they met weekly on Sundays. She had a sense of humour and made people happy. They were married in September.

After arriving in Burnley, Mackenzie was distressed by the living and working conditions of the majority of the population. Seeing much deep poverty he wrote a novel, Mary Helm, in which he related the tragedy of one working-class family, and described the social conditions of the industrial revolution and the early days of the Trade Union movement. Meanwhile, he continued to correspond with his family and friends.

Soon an awful event further stimulated his search for knowledge, an event described by McNair Wilson in "The Beloved Physician.[164] It was a case of prolonged childbirth to which MacKenzie was summoned one night.

"Let the reader imagine a room warm above the average, and cozy with screens set over against a cheerful fire... the anxious faces of old women, as a rule a midwife and a near relative of the young mother....

A great silence falls in the room. The girl's hair is wet with perspiration... her eyes glow in the lamplight. The doctor bends over and wipes her brow, supporting her with fresh assurances and encouragements....

Then comes a gentle knock at the door. The girl's mother, whose scarred old face is full of apprehension, rises and opens the door. It is the husband, who has come to ask if the ordeal will soon be ended.

"Yes, very soon."

"Is she all right, doctor?"

"Splendid."

"Thank God for that!"

The good fellow goes away comforted. The doctor returns to his post by the bedside.

"Was that John?"

"Yes. He's worrying about you."

"Poor old John!"

Again the silence possesses them... that strange, deep silence in which human souls arrive into this world, and in which also, as a rule, they depart from it. The doctor's mind, perhaps, is filled once again with the wonder which has so often filled it when he has seen the kindness and lovely courage of women during these supreme hours.

The girl's hand tightens its grip on his wrist, so that his thoughts are summoned sharply back to his duty. A dusky hue overspreads the glowing face beside him.

Suddenly the doctor starts from his chair. All the blood has run away from his cheeks. A wild fear shudders in his eyes.

He seizes the girl, and lifts her in his arms. His hands are set on her heart, as though they would compel it by force to resume its work... He pauses, glancing down at the fair young face. There is no colour now, and the long eyelashes fall in exquisite tranquillity on the cheeks.

"O God, can it be possible?"

He clutches at the wrists to feel the pulse.

The girl was dead. She had died of sudden heart failure. Neither did her baby survive. James Mackenzie, as he turned to break the news to her husband tasted the bitterest anguish which any doctor can ever experience.

Later, pacing in his consulting room through the silent hours of the night he faced the question, "would this death have occurred if I had had a better knowledge of heart afflictions?" He felt a sense of guilt that chilled his very soul.... His ignorance appalled him. He had examined this young woman carefully prior to her labour and had found no reason to expect difficulty at delivery.

From that moment he resolved to understand the function of the heart and its disorders, especially in pregnant women. Following that awful night Mackenzie became a dedicated researcher. Actually, he did not consider himself a researcher, he was too modest. He considered teaching hospitals to be the fount of research. He simply wanted to understand the heart's function and malfunction so that other patients would not die needlessly.

First, he searched the available literature, but found no help there. And so, he started to study his own patients and their hearts during pregnancy, both those with apparent heart damage and those apparently healthy. He noted the heart rate and any irregularities in its beat, its size and the presence and type of murmurs. He found that some of his patients with irregular heart beats experienced no difficulties during labour. The available books did not distinguish between the various irregularities. Which were dangerous? Mackenzie used a little instrument called a sphygmograph which could record each beat of the wrist pulse on moving paper. He discovered many differences in the size, form and rhythm of the waves produced. At first he could make little sense of them. Then he considered the veins in patients' necks, noting how some pulsated and others "fluttered like the wings of a bird." He was taught as a student that the throbbing of the neck veins was unimportant. Mackenzie venerated his teachers but felt he must investigate these throbbings further. But how to record them? He tried fixing a straw on the neck with gum to act as a pen and record a rather crude tracing on moving paper. Later he used a small funnel over the vein, the funnel being attached by a rubber tube to a thin rubber ball whose expansion and contraction he could record. He discovered three distinct waves in the neck veins which corresponded to specific events during the heart's contraction.

Using a more complex machine with a huge drum familiar to physiologists, he recorded the neck vein throbbings on one pen and the heart beat on another. He found that the second wave was caused by the nearby beating of the great carotid artery in the neck which followed the beating of the left ventricle or largest heart chamber, pushing the blood throughout the body. Wave No. 1 occurred just before wave No. 2 and corresponded to the beating of the right auricle which transferred blood from the great veins into the right ventricle which in turn passed the blood into the lungs. As the right auricle contracted, the increased pressure was partly transmitted back to neck veins, thus causing the first wave.

Mackenzie had found how to separate the action of the chambers of the heart. The nature of the third wave was obscure. He used to take his heavy apparatus into his patients' cottages, attach it to his patient and obtain a continuous record of their heart's contractions. Then, he smoked the strips in fumes of burning camphor to obtain a permanent record. Such a procedure provoked wonder among his patients. By making repeated tracings of his patients over the years, he was able to follow changes in their hearts. Not only was he able to learn of approaching danger, but could show, by 1900, that some irregularities such as occasional extra-systoles, (when the ventricle contracted prematurely before the auricle,) were relatively innocent.

Thus, he could reassure patients they could have a baby, perform heavy work or athletics without danger. His opinion differed from the prevalent teaching. Young people with occasional extra-systoles were often confined to bed for weeks.

I have described the extra-systole in rather simple terms. In Mackenzie's later work, <u>Diseases of the Heart</u>, first published in 1908, he described the extra-systole in 17 pages,[165] which some readers might wish to study. As for symptoms produced by extra-systoles, Mackenzie noted that most patients were unconscious of the condition until their attention was drawn to it, others were aware of the long pause "as if their heart had stopped;"[166] still others were aware of the following big beat. He continued to stress that in the absence of other symptoms there was no cause for alarm. He also demonstrated the innocence of what today is termed sinus arrhythmia, where the heart rate, especially in children, quickens during breathing in and slows while breathing out.

Mackenzie tried to pass his knowledge on to fellow doctors by writing articles for the more widely-read journals. However, their editors at first refused his work on the heart. Nevertheless he was satisfied to have "The significance of the pulsation in the veins," taken by the <u>Caledonian Medical Journal</u> in 1891; and, "A case of aneurysm of the heart with symptoms of angina pectoris during life," published by the <u>Manchester Medical Chronicle</u> that same year.

Ten years later the <u>British Medical Journal</u> published his observations on the heart irregularity occurring in a 40 year-old policeman with severe influenza.[167] While, in 1902 he published his findings in a book, The Study of the Pulse.[168] In the preface he quietly noted the circumstances in which he observed and wrote, ".... This volume has been written amid the distractions of the life of a busy general practitioner... I have seldom been able to give an uninterrupted hour's study to the subject. While working out some argument... it has been days and even weeks before I have been able to resume it...." [169]

Apart from the volume of patients he saw at their homes or in his "surgery," he delivered many maternity cases each year. His industry was phenomenal. He tried to write a little first thing in the morning, then again in the evening, when he wrote up his notes while enjoying his wife's piano playing in the background. Frances learned how to type and managed to interpret his scrawled handwriting for publication.

The couple had two daughters whom they loved dearly. Sadly, the eldest developed polio and permanent paralysis of her left leg at 17 months while their younger daughter died of meningitis when sixteen years old.

Slowly recognition came to Mackenzie; at first, mostly from abroad. For example, the Dutch researcher, Wenckebach, read Mackenzie's Study of the Pulse and some of his papers. A steady correspondence followed.

Frequently, they agreed on many points, and Mackenzie visited Wenckebach at the University of Groningen in 1904. Meanwhile, about 1903, the anatomist Arthur Keith became fascinated by Mackenzie's observations and was able to dissect the hearts of Mackenzie's dead patients, finding them to be "the only specimens to have full pre-mortem records.[170] (My underlining.) In one of his notebooks, Mackenzie described a Mrs. Ashworth with shortness of breath whom he first examined in May 1892. She experienced frequent ventricular extra-systoles. She happened to be the first patient in whom he was able to demonstrate that the extra-systoles were due to premature contraction of the ventricle. She died 15 years later and Keith performed the autopsy, finding great dilation of the auricles and degenerative changes in the auriculo-ventricular bundle, (the fibres which transmit the heart beat.) The artery supplying blood and oxygen to the bundle was greatly thickened and minute vessels closed.[171]

The pathological examination explained the patient's clinical findings during life. As Canadian researcher Dr. William Gibson, (under whom I did research for one year at the University of B.C.) wrote,[172]

"Most of all, Mackenzie proved for all eyes to see, that clinical science was a field crying out to be studied.... When Osler went from Johns Hopkins to become Regius Professor at Oxford in 1905, he lost no time in visiting Mackenzie in Burnley as Cushing records, with A.G. Gibson from the Radcliffe Infirmary. A year later Sir Arthur Hurst returned from Germany to blast his British colleagues with the startling information that only Mackenzie was known on the continent. Thus did a general practitioner, working quietly but purposefully for thirty years in a Lancashire mill town with the people he loved build the framework upon which all scientific cardiology rests today."

In the social conditions of Burnley and of course long before the discovery of penicillin, Mackenzie followed many patients who had developed complications following rheumatic fever such as narrowing of heart valves or damage to its conducting system causing an irregular heart beat. He used the term "auricular paralysis' to describe the weak erratic beats which sometimes occurred in the auricles and is today known as auricular fibrillation.' He also followed Withering in using digitalis, finding that digitalis would slow the ventricular rate of the heart and relieve heart failure.[173]

Mackenzie carefully described angina pectoris.[174] He emphasized the heart was a muscle which, when exhausted, could produce an attack of angina. The exhaustion could follow many activities. "The heart is", he would say, "as the heart does." A sign or symptom was only significant in so far as its presence indicated the onset of heart failure. It was important to listen to the patient to learn from his tale what brought on the attack and to avoid that activity. Examining patients with angina he often found no abnormality. The story was central to the diagnosis. Interestingly, he commented, "The attack of pain may not come for some minutes or even hours after the causal exertion has ceased...."

He noted the distribution of skin hypersensitivity on the left arm which sometimes accompanied or followed an attack of angina. One patient described feeding himself with his right hand, because moving his left arm sometimes initiated an attack. Mackenzie was to learn the nature of angina pectoris only too well as it so affected his final years. He warned patients not to overindulge in tobacco. He continued to appreciate the help of anatomist Arthur Keith in linking pathological findings with his patient's symptoms during life.

At fifty-four years of age, Mackenzie, after much thought, decided to leave his steady practice in Burnley to begin again in London. The first year was disastrous. From being incredibly busy he hardly saw a patient. They became poor. Their youngest daughter died. Having much spare time he finished the final copy of his great work, <u>Diseases of the Heart</u>. This work brought him a reasonable income, patients and more recognition. Despite having no FRCP he was offered an appointment as Physician to the West London Hospital and advised by a medical friend to move into world famous Harley Street. <u>Diseases of the Heart</u> was full of his observations and research, and was of real practical value to other doctors.

Following his own advice that 'the heart is as the heart does,' he encouraged patients to gradually undertake exercises which would not cause significant shortness of breath or pain. For example, one 68 year-old patient who had been dissuaded by two distinguished physicians to avoid all activity because of auricular fibrillation was enabled to return to regular activities, walking two miles a day, and cycling which he loved. His improvement continued during the next seven years in which he was able to keep in touch.[175]

Soon Mackenzie was invited to become a lecturer on cardiac research at the London Hospital with six beds at his disposal. In 1915 he was made a Fellow of the Royal Society. During World War I his opinion was sought about cases of "soldier's heart." He used exercise as the major therapeutic aid.

Mackenzie never considered himself to be a heart specialist. He looked upon himself as still a general practitioner, also acting as a consultant. He felt that general practice was the best place to see the earliest signs of illness and a valuable research opportunity.

While at the height of his career, fame and fortune he astounded everyone by giving up his London practice and returning to general practice to share his knowledge with other practitioners and with students. This he did at the St. Andrews Institute in Scotland from 1919 till 1924 when severe angina forced his retirement. His life ended after he had just completed proofs for a new edition of Diseases of the Heart, rather as Anton Chekhov died after completing The Cherry Orchard.

Mackenzie always stressed the importance of the patient's tale and examination findings more than any diagnostic machine. His research always aimed to benefit the patient. He tried to encourage other practitioners to start research in their practices, but few followed his lead. Commenting on today's research in general practice, J.R. Howie from Edinburgh stated that too often research "seems to be pursuing a managerial rather than a clinician's agenda, and certainly not a patient's agenda."[176]

Mair concluded, "Today, the problems of morbidity in general practice may differ but they still exist and for their elucidation await a modern Mackenzie armed not with expensive and electronic equipment but with intuitive and instructive powers of observation, capacity for hard work and determination to succeed."[177]

15

SOME CANADIAN PHYSICIANS

It is difficult to choose from among the many doctors who served Canadians during the 20th century. I shall limit the present chapter to Canadian general practitioners working in their regular practices outside the life of the university. In chapter three we noted Abraham Groves, the country doctor from Fergus, Ontario, who in 1883 performed the first successful appendectomy in North America.[14]

For balance I will choose one other doctor from eastern Canada and two from the western provinces. Their work is important and it reveals a more complete tale of medical research and care. Furthermore, the illustrious Anton Chekhov wrote of "little writers"... "The lower ranks are just as indispensable in literature as they are in the army."[178]

EDMUND A. BRASSET (1910-1963)

Becoming a general practitioner was furthest from the mind of young Dalhousie medical student, Edmund Brasset. Brasset was fired with enthusiasm for the human brain and aspired to a much higher "caste" as he put it in his autobiography.[179] His ambition was to become a brain surgeon.

And so in his final student year he studied night and day, having little time to spend with a certain hazel-eyed nurse Sally MacNeil. His work and self-discipline proved all in vain, for the Dean of Medicine informed him at the end of the year that he would not be recommended for the desired residency.

It was 1933, and there was little money available toward the end of the depression. Brasset, depressed at having to become a lowly G.P. and having absorbed from his medical teachers that such doctors while not quite buffoons were certainly second rate, drove the rocky road to start practice in the isolated coastal town of Canso in Nova Scotia. I have chosen two excerpts from his autobiography. The first tale concerns the very first patient Brassett treated in Canso.[180]

I was still unpacking my equipment the next morning when I had my first patient. A woman of about thirty years of age, who looked as if she were forty, came to the office carrying a small, thin and sickly infant in her arms.

"I don't know what to do with him," she told me, with a wan and helpless expression. "He don't seem to be gaining any and he cries all the time."

"What kind of formula are you giving him?" I asked her.

"Formula!" she repeated in a puzzled tone.

"The milk," I said. "How much do you give him and how do you mix it?"

"We don't give him no milk at all." She obviously considered my question very odd. "After all he's four months old."

I looked at her in surprise. "You don't give him milk!" I exclaimed, "Why not? What do you give him then?"

"There ain't no milk," she answered. "There's not even one cow in Alewife Point where we live. You don't expect us to buy canned milk, do you?"

I did not know what to say, so I repeated, "Then what do you give him?"

"Fish, of course," she replied, "what else! Dry cod. I grate it up and he kind of chews it, although he ain't got any teeth yet, and swallows it. And of course he gets bread and molasses too. Molasses is very good for babies. Sometimes we give him a little tea."

"Fish and tea at four months?"

"Sure, the tea is strengthening. Sometimes I stir a little flour into the tea to give it body like. That's strengthening too and besides it makes the bones stick together good."

Fish and tea and flour for a baby of four months! I thought for a while and then I wrote out a formula for the baby consisting of evaporated milk, corn syrup and water. She was not satisfied.

"Aren't you going to give him any medicine?" she asked.

"All the medicine he needs is proper food," I said, "and don't give him any more dry cod and tea."

She still looked doubtful but she went away. This, I learned, was a pretty general way of feeding babies in the area. The reason for the lack of cows was the lack of fodder, for there was hardly any space for grass to grow between the rocks.... The people had for so long been accustomed to taking their living from the sea that they did not readily learn anything pertaining to farming for, with a few exceptions, there is a point at which poverty takes away even the will to escape from poverty....

A week or so later I called in to see Alex Doran, the storekeeper to whom I had sent the woman. I asked him for the bill.

"Four eighty, Doc."

I paid him and then he said, "Do you know what happened to that case of milk?"

"No," I said, "but I hope the baby is drinking it. Why do you ask?"

"Oh, nothing," he said, "only the day after I gave them the case, she came in here and bought a new yellow scarf. One of those in that show case there, for a dollar and a half, and that's not all. That same afternoon, Pete Smith came in and offered to sell me a case of milk. Told me he'd take three dollars for it. I bought it–here it is here."

"You mean she sold the milk to Pete Smith and bought a new scarf!" I yelped.

"That's right, Doc." He looked at me shrewdly and then he laughed.

"Give it up, Doc," he urged,

Curiously, the baby recovered.

'It was fifteen below zero one evening when, just at dusk, Johnny Hall and I climbed into his open sleigh and started out for White Harbour, thirty-five miles and ten hours away.[181]

Fifteen below zero, in a place near the sea, is very cold indeed. We both wore fur coats and were dressed as warmly as we could manage, but were not equipped like those people who inhabit the extreme north and who have to contend with the severest climate nine months of the year. After the first hour out, we felt that the expression "chilled to the bone" had a very literal meaning. I could picture little crystals of ice in my spinal fluid. I said to Johnny, "Is it possible to get any colder than this!"

"Sure is cold," he answered. He was a good man, but not one to talk much. During the next two hours we tried getting out and walking up the hills. This helped a little, but could not be kept up for long because of the slippery ice in some places and the heavy snow in others. Moreover, after the exertion of walking we seemed to be colder than ever as soon as we sat in the sleigh again. During the last two hours both of us, I think, were a little delirious from the cold. I cursed the day when I had taken up the study of medicine. I remember having bitter thoughts too, about the patient we were going to see. There would be nothing wrong with him except a slight cold. He was probably sitting up at this very minute alongside a hot stove, drinking rum and hot water and laughing to himself at how he was making a fool of the new doctor. He would, of course, not pay me–almost no one ever did on these trips even though they might have the money cached in a tin box under the bed–but would promise to pay as soon as his cheque came in. All of a sudden, with all my heart I hated this patient whom I had never seen. I hated the country and I hated my own profession most of all.

Finally we arrived at the small house where the patient lay. As soon as I saw him, I forgot all about hating him. He was a very sick man and he was in extreme pain. I knew what was wrong with him before I got near the bed and before I heard a word of his story. He had acute urinary retention. There are very few conditions that can be more distressing than this. Also it can be usually very quickly and easily relieved... I huddled over the stove in an attempt to get warm. The woman gave us hot tea and after a little while I began to get thawed out.

Sterilising the instruments took about twenty minutes and all the time the man on the bed was writhing and groaning aloud. I could not begin to help him until my hands were thawed out.'

Dr. Brasset tried to pass a catheter to allow the man's urine to flow out, but he was unsuccessful. Then he learned that the patient had needed to have a cystostomy done during a prior retention. (An opening made through the abdominal and bladder wall.) The only thing to do now was to operate upon the man just where he lay....

The operation under local anaesthesia, although it involves a three inch incision through the lower part of the abdomen and a smaller one through the bladder, is a simple one and it did not take long to do.

In a little while the wound was closed with a rubber drain securely in place. The transformation in the patient was something to see. He actually cried with relief and joy, and in a little while was sleeping the quiet sleep of exhaustion.

The woman gave me another cup of hot tea. As I drank it and smoked a cigarette I thought, "So what if I get paid with an imaginary cheque, and I have to pay Johnny Hall with real dollars, and if there are lots of comfortable easy jobs with regular hours? This is worth doing!"

On the way home Brasset developed a sense of lightness, as if he had got rid of some heavy burden when he realised that the Mayo brothers with all their skill and all their facilities could not have done what he had done for this patient. They were in Minnesota, two thousand miles away. They might have been on the moon as far as the people of Canso were concerned. Somehow he had overlooked this simple fact.

Dr. Brasset's autobiography well reveals the perplexities, the pathos, the humour and the triumphs of a country practice. Unfortunately, he found himself going ever deeper into debt. After marrying the hazel-eyed Sally MacNeil, he worked in a mental hospital where they received room, board and a steady income. Later when he relocated to Little Brook, Nova Scotia, and was actually paid for his services by his patients he finally earned enough to enter a residency in his chosen specialty of neurosurgery. However, in the rather sterile hospital wards he found that he missed the close relationship with his patients and returned to his country practice with a settled mind.

Mary Percy Jackson (1905-2000)

Travelling west across Canada, we come to the province of Alberta where Dr. Mary Jackson joined a travelling medical clinic started by the Alberta Government after World War I to care for the fresh wave of immigrants (mostly of European or British extraction) as well as the native Indians living in the remote communities.

Women doctors were rare in those days, but four pioneering women joined the clinic. Some believe that country doctors were not trained thoroughly, but one of these women, Dr. Margaret Owens, had delivered eight hundred babies during her training, while Dr. Mary Jackson won the prize for highest marks in medicine, surgery and midwifery in her 1927 class at the University of Birmingham in England, and had pursued extra training in medicine, surgery, paediatrics, obstetrics and anaesthesia, so she was well qualified to deal with the wide variety of conditions in a pioneer setting.

She had another important talent, she was a competent horsewoman.

She answered an Alberta government advertisement for women doctors who were able to live and work alone, without access to hospital facilities, treating whatever happened in remote areas–and the ability to ride a saddle would be an advantage.

Soon she found herself rattling in the train for a week, mile after mile across the nearly uninhabited country from Quebec to Edmonton, and then North to the Peace River area. She described some of her experiences to Henri Chatenay who wrote The <u>Country Doctors</u>.[182]

'When I got to Battle River Landing I got my luggage loaded on a wagon by a morose Indian who couldn't speak a word of English, and his little team of cayuses couldn't pull the wagon up the hill. So we had to unload the stuff and carry it. Eventually we arrived at the cabin where we would live.

The cabin was locked and there was no key. It was evening and the mosquitoes were biting like mad. There was a bridge crew, building a bridge across the First Battle or Notikewin River, and they gave us a sandwich we needed badly. Somebody got a key and we got into the cabin, which was dirty, and the water bucket had a hole in it. To get water, you had to go down to the river and by the time you got to the top of the bank, there wasn't much water left in the pail. There were a few black-handled knives and forks, a few dishes and a bed. I did bring some flower vases and ornaments. A few, because you don't carry a vast amount of stuff when you are going into the bush, and I had little in the way of personal stuff. Some books –Osler's Text book of Medicine which I had been brought up on, Gray's Anatomy, Williams's Obstetrics – that told of the dreadful things that could happen. It was worth keeping a hundred books on the off-chance that you needed one desperately. I kept buying new books all the time.

You treated "by guess and by God" and hoped that things would go right. There was a steady stream of odd cases – babies, axe wounds, and fractures were the main things. People didn't go in much for neurotic illness in those days. For one thing, they were a 'selected' population. They were the people who'd gone homesteading. Anybody who was too nervous about being isolated, just didn't go, so they were a fitter than average population. A large number were Central Europeans – Poles and Ukrainians – who weren't used to being doctored. The Indians, of course, had never been doctored, so they didn't come around with minor ailments.

It makes a vast difference when people are living an interesting and demanding existence like homesteading. So you've got to get a roof over your head when the snow comes. You've got to get the potatoes in the cellar before winter comes. And you've got access to no help except that of your own neighbours. Therefore, you don't have time to think of your ailments. When they were sick – they were very sick. This was all before antibiotics or sulpha drugs. Fevers were high and the people who were sick depended on their own powers of recovery. There wasn't a vast amount that the doctor could do for them. But fractures and accidents, knife and axe wounds you could do something about. If they went septic, you had problems, because the long fight with severely infected wounds was a problem. This is where a man called Barron Rose, who taught me surgery, had hammered into me, with much in the way of strong language, that the correct way to cope with dirty wounds was to remove the dirty muscle until you got down to good clean muscle – which was useful information – when you got stuck with somebody who'd been dragged two miles by a horse after their foot had got caught in the stirrup – what you knew about cleaning dirty wounds came in very handy...."

They brought me a lot of patients because that was quicker than sending somebody to fetch me. There was no phone – there was no way of getting word to the doctor – so the patients tried to come if they possibly could. Maternity cases and pneumonia, of course, I had to go out on.

When people were very ill and dying of tuberculosis – you could not get them into the San, so they stayed home and infected the rest of the family before they died. They used to sing and their singing certainly helped the patient more than my medicine would have done. What could I give them? Aspirin. We had aspirin in those days....'[182]

After working two years for the clinic she married Frank Jackson who farmed the northern Peace River County at Keg River. There as a farmer's wife she was still in heavy demand as a doctor in that isolated community for 43 years.

'When I first came to Keg River the Indian Medicine Man was quite a friend. He'd lost one lung to tuberculosis and he's one of the few people that I've ever heard of who had what we call, Hippocratic succussion. If you shook him, you could hear a splash in the huge abscess in his chest.

He called me when he was sick one time. He'd drunk a whole case of Wampole's Extract of Cod Liver Oil, which was the medicine that was sold in large quantities by the traders in the early days – more for its alcoholic content than its Cod Liver Oil. It came in pint bottles and, as I remember, twelve bottles to the case. There was a small amount of strychnine in it and we used strychnine as a tonic in those days. Anyway, the dose being two teaspoonfuls, the effect of drinking twelve pint bottles one after another gave him strychnine poisoning as well as alcohol poisoning At first I thought he might have tetanus. When

I'd found out what he had been doing, I decided he had strychnine poisoning. Anyway, the only thing I could think of to do was to give him a powerful laxative, because I thought that whatever this stuff was it was still in his gut and we'd better get rid of it. He recovered all right and he said that I'd found the right thing to make him move. He had to move – because no Indian will ever use a toilet pail in the house. They always go out even when they're dying of pneumonia. So this old man had to keep running to the outside privy and he figured that cured him. He thought it was a great joke!'

'In 1931 this Polish woman was having what is known as occipital posterior presentation or "deep transverse arrest of the head." She'd been in strong labour for three days and was getting exhausted, before her husband realised that she was not just having a baby, which every woman was expected to do in Poland without the benefit of doctoring. He probably didn't know that there was a doctor available in the Battle River district. If he did he had no way of getting to me easily as he had only one horse and a sort of a toboggan. So he got a neighbour to fetch me. This man was living in a little cabin built of poplar poles, with straw on the roof. His cow and horse were in a lean-to, and in the part that they were in, the poles weren't chinked between that and the house. The cabin had no windows but there was a little square of glass in the door.

There were two families living in the cabin. There was a mud floor and the woman's bed was a wooden shelf, – attached to the wall – with one bedpost at the corner. The other corners, of course, were on the wall. The pigs and chickens were under the bed – I don't remember how many pigs – two or three anyway. There was one stove and the woman, of the other family, was busy cooking. The interpreter I had couldn't speak her language very well. I had to get the fetus head back in the womb and turned around before I could put the forceps on it to deliver it – without anybody to give the anaesthetic that I could talk to – without any assistance – with pigs nuzzling at my feet from under the bed – and without proper light. But the woman and the baby survived and I seem to remember that the baby weighed nine pounds. Meanwhile, the other woman was busy frying potatoes in the grease on the stove and she wasn't too careful, because the grease caught fire and there were flames shooting into the straw on the ceiling – just the straw that you could see between the poles that made the roof. It was quite exciting!'

Mary Jackson described her adventures to writer Henri Chatenay who authored the account.[182] As she lived a full life as pioneer and farmer's wife, giving birth to five children, dealing with seriously ill patients, and often riding long hours in the saddle, she did not have much time for writing. She lived to the age of ninety-five.

C. CHAN GUNN (1931 -)

Some readers may not appreciate that besides providing valuable care Brasset and Jackson also performed basic observational research into the social conditions of their communities. Another G.P./family doctor to do so was 1988 University of British Columbia graduate Harvey Thommasen who researched the natural history of the Bella Coola Valley, home of the river which reaches the Pacific Ocean at Bella Coola, British Columbia.

'He'd captured and identified hundreds of aquatic insects, memorised sound tapes so that he could recognise birds by their songs, done clinical studies on Native medicinal plants and taken time out of his rounds to question elders about the way things had been.'[183]

He provided the basic field notes for writer/fisherman Mark Hume to produce River of the Angry Moon, describing the passing of the seasons, the natives, the fishing and the near destruction of a beautiful river through our continuing greed and folly.[184]

But another type of pain is the major problem that confronts patients and their physicians; the problem we saw earlier which concerned James Mackenzie, and it was another B.C. doctor, Dr. C. Chan Gunn, born in Malaysia in 1931 who researched pain during the last quarter of the 20th century and continues to do so into the 21st century.

In October 2001 Dr. Gunn kindly invited me to see his work. He impressed me immediately by his thorough examination of patients, by his consideration for them, and by the very difficult pain problems he was asked to evaluate and help. Despite many long histories of pain and treatment including surgical procedures, he helped most patients significantly. His enthusiasm was infectious. He told me of his experiences and training and taught me his basic method.

He had studied Natural Sciences at Peterhouse, Cambridge University after the war in Malaysia when he and his Chinese family were fortunate to survive terrible hardships during the Japanese invasion of their country.

After clinical experience at University College Hospital in London and passing his examinations, he began two years of post graduate work, first in Epsom hospital, where he studied general surgery and orthopaedics. Next he studied paediatrics at Paddington Green Childrens' Hospital under Dr. Thomas Stapleton. It was there working with many malnourished children in the Paddington area that he showed in his first published paper how anaemic infants responded to treatment with ferrous fumarate, an iron preparation more easily taken by his small patients than ferrous sulphate.[185] He also wrote on cretinism.

At further hospital posts he spent extra time in medicine, obstetrics, gynaecology and ear, nose and throat. Working in non-teaching hospitals with less staff he had to perform much laboratory work and take x-rays, tasks he made use of later. Meanwhile he married Peggy Loke, an accomplished artist who was studying architecture in London. They had a son and daughter. In 1958 they left for Malaysia where he started a general practice in his own country. Just before leaving he happened to be given some samples of an antibiotic furodantin which were to prove most valuable.

In the early days of his own practice a wealthy patient, Mr. Ng consulted him for a second opinion. He had been undergoing hospital treatment for a serious kidney infection, diabetes, a grave leg ulcer, and had been advised to have his leg amputated. Gunn gave Mr. Ng the furodantin he had obtained in England and cleared up the kidney infection. The patient's diabetes and leg ulcer also improved under Gunn's care. The patient spread the news of his cure widely, helping Gunn develop a successful practice in which he also did much of his own laboratory work, took his own x-rays and produced medication for his patients at little or no cost.

In 1966 he emigrated to Canada, briefly researching at the University of British Columbia. Next he joined the Workers' Compensation Board where he found the opportunity to study persisting pain.

Low back pain was and is a major problem among workers attending the Compensation Board. For example, in 1974 one third of all admissions were due to low back injuries.[186] Of these 86 percent were given the "working diagnosis" of low-back sprain. The remainder had fractures or prior back surgery.

Gunn found that some of these back sprain patients had tender points in some muscles, (known as motor points) which revealed abnormal electromyographic findings. Palpating carefully he discovered these points to be consistent anatomically. For example, he found that a small tender area in the upper outer quadrant of the buttock, previously attributed to "gluteal bursitis" was simply a tender motor point in the gluteal medius muscle.

The tender motor points were located in the myotomes corresponding to the probable segmental levels of spinal injury and root involvement. Examining fifty patients with low-back sprain, Gunn found 26 to have tender motor points. In contrast, only seven control patients revealed minor motor point tenderness following strenuous activity. Gunn noted that patients with low-back sprain and no tender motor points were disabled an average of 6.9 weeks, those with tender motor points 19.7 weeks, and those with nerve root involvement 25.7 weeks. The tender motor points were therefore of both diagnostic and prognostic importance.[186]

Next, he turned his attention to "tennis elbow" and its possible connection with the cervical spine.[187] In a series of 37 men and 13 women patients referred to the WCB rehabilitation centre and who had received varying treatments to their elbows without benefit, he found tender motor points in the extensor muscles of the wrist and some abnormal electromyographic findings suggesting early nerve or nerve root damage. Applying physical treatment including traction and mobilisation to the neck rather than the elbow he obtained satisfactory relief of elbow symptoms in 86 percent of patients after five weeks of therapy.[187]

While examining his low back sprain patients Gunn had noted subtle abnormalities related to denervation, consisting of autonomic dysfunction, trophic changes, hypersensitivity and increased muscle tone. The changes were familiar to physiologists and to clinicians treating patients with peripheral nerve injuries, but not familiar to those examining patients with low back pain.[188] He noted anatomic dysfunction when patients undressed exposing their skin to cool air which led to developing "goose flesh" in the affected dermatone and sometimes mottling of the skin following constriction of small blood vessels. Also, he noted abnormal sweating.

Furthermore, skin and underlying subcutaneous tissue might become "boggy" or trophedematous. Pressing the blunt end of a match-stick into the skin Gunn demonstrated boggyness by the pitting of the skin. By careful palpation he also demonstrated increased sensitivity and muscle tone.[189]

Meanwhile, he had studied traditional acupuncture but found it largely non-scientific. Nevertheless, some traditional acupuncture points corresponded to his tender motor points in specific muscles. Using acupuncture needles he needled the points he had discovered on clinical examination and found such technique effective in 29 male low back pain patients at the WCB compared with 27 "control" subjects.[190] Lewit also reported the beneficial effect of dry needling in myofascial pain.[191]

Next, Gunn came across the long neglected work of Cannon and Rosenblueth in their 1949 study The Supersensitivity of Denervated Structures.[192] Walter Cannon was Professor of Physiology at Harvard University in the 1940's and had died prior to the publication of their work which curiously attracted little interest.

Cannon stated,[192] "when in a series of efferent neurons a unit is destroyed, an increased irritability to chemical agents develops in the isolated structure or structures, the effects being maximal in the part directly denervated." Supersensitivity develops not only in striated muscle but also in other structures such as smooth muscle, sweat glands, autonomic ganglion cells, spinal neurons and even brain cells.

Gunn summarised Cannon's work and other related experiments in a 1980 review paper in Spine,[193] and later in his own practical text, The Gunn Approach to the Treatment of Chronic Pain.[194]

He used the term neuropathy to describe dysfunction in the peripheral nervous system recognised by Cannon.Neuropathy causes increased muscle tone and muscle shortening which in turn causes a wide variety of pain syndromes by its relentless pull on various structures. Muscle shortening is the "key to myofascial pain of neuropathic origin."[195] Muscle shortening can be palpated as ropy bands within muscle. Shortening in paraspinal muscles acting across an intervertebral disc may compress the disc and narrow the intervertebral foramina, irritating the nerve root and causing its dysfunction.

Having located the area of muscle shortening, Gunn then uses traditional acupuncture needles to penetrate that specific point, the motor point. When entering normal muscle the needle encounters minimal resistance, but on penetrating the affected site, the needle encounters marked resistance and is grasped by spasm in the muscle. The patient experiences a cramp-like sensation, sometimes quite severe, known to traditional acupuncturists as the DEQI phenomenon. Such sensation confirms the needle is placed correctly. The needle is then moved by small jabs, "pecking" the tissue thoroughly. The needle is then left in place and the spasm relaxes in about five minutes. Nearby sites are then treated similarly. Concurrent electrical stimulation may be used. The needle itself causes minute local tissue damage and release of the Platelet Derived Growth Factor which promotes mitosis and healing. The needle injury also causes an electrical current which promotes continuing relief of spasm. Frequently the needling also causes some relaxation in nearby muscles. Its prolonging effect makes the technique far superior to commonly used physiotheraputic techniques such as TENS. Examining the patient later, an increased range of movement in the affected muscle groups can be demonstrated. Gunn terms his technique intramuscular stimulation or IMS.

IMS is remarkably safe compared to many other remedies. The fine point needle has no cutting edge. To use the technique a practitioner needs a thorough knowledge of anatomy and physiology and adequate training which Dr. Gunn and his associates offer at his Institute for the Study and Treatment of Pain at Vancouver, British Columbia, Canada. Physicians and physiotherapists are especially suited for his training programs.

Local recognition has come slowly to Dr. Gunn. Some have confused his work with acupuncture. Nevertheless in 1983 he was invited to join the University of Washington Multidisciplinary Pain Centre as a consultant.[196] Dr. Patrick Wall, in his foreword to Dr. Gunn's text,[197] pointed out that it was "in the best tradition of classical medicine," that it was in no way "complementary" or "alternative medicine," but was based upon classic anatomy, physiology and pathology. Wall noted that his work "requires a meticulous hands-on clinical examination of the individual patient... a lost art in favour of supposedly effective high-tech methods.... It requires subtle sensitive empirical treatment of the individual patient."

"It is true that he characterises the precise nature of the disorders in terms of neuropathies and compressions, but these are hypotheses which are permissible because they are testable by accepted methods of investigation. Almost all traditional medical diagnoses are based upon hypotheses which have not yet been fully tested and proven."[197]

Dr. Gunn is invited to demonstrate his work in many countries. He has attracted the attention of many high quality practitioners from North America and overseas, some of whom I have had the pleasure of meeting.

He was awarded a rare Honorary Fellowship at Peterhouse in Cambridge, and in 2002 received the Order of Canada for his services to medicine and to the community. He and his wife Peggy are strong supporters of the arts and Dr. Gunn was founding director of the Canadian Society for Asian Art. Truly, he has built a bridge between East and West.

Recently, Dr. Gunn and his associates treated me for a long standing lumbar disc problem. I found the treatment while not comfortable to be most effective. I wish I had learned from him earlier.

Dr. Gunn has accomplished a remarkable volume of original work. Until the 1970s, medical diagnosis generally considered pain to result from tissue injury. However, Dr. Gunn's clinical research showed that pain can occur without injury when there is abnormal function of the nervous system. His innovative concept of "neuropathic pain" has led to significant changes in the understanding and treatment of chronic pain.

He has completed some 30 or more scientific articles and books, and has clearly demonstrated that a family physician today can through perseverance still contribute significantly to medical research just as James Mackenzie did a century ago. Contemporary family doctors should test Gunn's work for themselves and explore research opportunities in their own practices. If you have not heard of Dr. Chan Gunn, here is a good example of little known medical research by a family doctor.

Listening to these tales from the past broadens our understanding of medicine.

We need research and we need heroes.

16

Do Not Forget

During the introduction (vi) we noted the importance of the tale to medicine and in the first two sections provided numerous examples of patients' tales and their value in recording history and diagnoses. We noted tales from parts of Canada and elsewhere. It seems appropriate to close with a tale describing an incident among first nations people on one of the islands off the west coast of British Columbia.

I was exchanging stories with another west coast doctor whom I met during a medical meeting one fall. Bearded and broad-shouldered Johann would have pulled an oar with ease. Currently his strong hands enveloped a tankard of beer.

"It's strange", he remarked, "how grateful some people are."

"Cathie and I have a little place on Narvaez island. It's just a shack, really, but we go there with our son Jim in the summer to get away from the rat race."

I could picture him there in the setting sun, leaning against the hut, his boy chasing their dog and maybe a freshly-caught salmon lying in the grass by his feet.

"Two years ago", he continued, "there was a serious car accident on the island. We have only two roads, but where they meet an old car had smashed into a truck. I must have arrived moments after the crash. There were two first nation's boys in the car. One had been thrown out on the edge of the road. He was lying there groaning and one of his legs was badly bent. It was obviously broken but he wasn't in serious danger.

The other kid was quiet, jammed against the wheel, not breathing. I dragged him out with difficulty." Johann moved his hands expressively. "He was unconscious; so I laid him on the ground and started resuscitation."

Johann paused to sip his beer. I could see him kneeling by the car, his great frame bent over the quiet boy, mouth applied to the boy's mouth, breathing for him, giving him life, then pushing on his chest with those strong hands, compressing the heart and lungs, pushing the oxygenated blood back to the brain and the vital organs.

"I worked on him for about ten minutes. By this time his heart had restarted, he was breathing on his own and colour was coming back into his cheeks."

"Meanwhile the truck driver watched from a distance, leaning against his truck, saying nothing, just looking. The other boy still groaned by the side of the road. I turned the first boy onto his side and made a rough splint for the groaning boy. Then the police arrived and radioed for a helicopter. Two hours later both kids were recovering in the big city hospital. However the boy jammed against the wheel was left with some weakness in his arm...."

"Next summer, we returned to Narvaez island. We arrived on the ferry and spent an hour visiting with friends. When we reached the cabin we were surprised to find fruit, vegetables and two silver salmon on the porch. How did the people know we had arrived?

And fruit, vegetables or salmon kept coming. The people offered to do any work on the place. How many would have responded that way? How many city folk?

I did not reply.

"Even next year some gifts still came - as reliably as a flowing tide."

I looked at those hands and saw again the dusty road, the boy, the rhythm of hands on chest, mouth on mouth, life to life, the folk with gifts.

Johann placed his tankard on the table and leaned forward more earnestly, commanding my attention.

"Those people, they love or they hate. They do not forget."

More Researching

17

CLOSER TO HOME

Despite the accomplishments of those physicians noted in the previous section, and others since, general practice, often termed family medicine today, still remains the most unresearched field in medicine. Even James Mackenzie felt that research took place at the teaching hospital and was essentially beyond his reach.[154] Surely his career proved otherwise.

In 1972, country doctor William Pickles declared,[146]

"...I have known several country practitioners with useful knowledge to impart, gathered from their own observations, but who considered it too trivial even to write down, much less to publish. Nothing I believe is further from the truth, and by withholding these observations from the public, these men are damming up sources of information that are among the only accurate ones from which such information can be drawn."

So it may prove useful to contemporary students and practitioners and even those outside medicine if I record a little of my experiences and of my background.

I never dreamt of doing research, I started quite by mistake having been struck by ideas which surfaced during some post-graduate study and regular practice. Previously, just prior to World War II and during that conflict, my father had performed vital research in night vision.

A distinguished eye specialist, he was born at Cowichan Bay, Vancouver Island, B.C. Canada in 1893. Far behind academically he "crammed" at a London coaching "college", and squeezed into Cambridge University to study medicine in 1912.[198]

He was motivated to study hard but was persuaded to row for his college and in 1914 was chosen to row for Cambridge against Oxford, becoming the first Canadian to obtain his rowing "blue."

After wartime service and qualifying at the London hospital he joined the young Royal Air Force and for a few years performed essentially general practice overseas. Partly due to ill health he later specialized in ophthalmology, and in 1934 was appointed head of the RAF medical services eye department.

In 1937 the Air Council sent him to Germany where he had the opportunity to observe the excellent research being conducted by Luftwaffe doctors. The Germans were well ahead of the RAF and were obviously preparing for war.[199] Nevertheless, they were not researching night vision, intending to fly, fight and bomb during the day. On his return to England my father sent a detailed account of his observations on German achievements and war preparations which greatly interested the Air Council. Then he laboured to improve visual standards among RAF personnel, researching the effects on vision of diminished oxygen at high altitudes, inventing an improved goggle for air crew, and investigating night vision.

He found that pilots with good day vision might see quite poorly at night due to deficient rod cells in the retina and invented a machine, the rotating hexagon, to discover those best suited for night flying.[200] After the Battle of Britain the Germans switched mostly to night bombing. British night fighters with excellent night vision saw the enemy first and shot down aircraft before German rear-gunners could see them. It took the Germans a year to discover why. My father's night vision research had a significant effect on the outcome of the war.

He seemed to write his scientific articles with ease and also his autobiography, <u>Fringe of the Clouds</u>, published in 1962.[198]

However, writing never came naturally to me. In 1954, having graduated from the University of Alberta, interned there and done two extra valuable months training in anesthesia under Dr. Gain in Edmonton, I started medical practice with the excellent firm of Drs Hall, Giovando, Blott and Philcox in Nanaimo, B.C. They taught me a great deal.

Next, I spent a year with Dr. Bill Gibson doing neurological research at the University of British Columbia and then a year at St. Paul's hospital studying orthopedics under Dr. Arthur McConkey, and general surgery. That year I met and spent much time with New Zealander Diana Berkeley. We married in September and set up practice in agricultural Richmond, also a bedroom community for Vancouver at the Fraser river delta.

After a few years of solo medical practice I happened to attend a continuing medical education lecture on spinal manipulation at St. Vincent's hospital in Vancouver, an experience described in chapter six. The lecturer, heavy set orthopedic surgeon Gerald Burke, later invited me to see his work. Practising under his direction I found I could help some of my back and neck pain patients more and began to have patients referred to me by other doctors. Meanwhile I learned from James Cyriax, (England), John Andrews, John Mennell, Janet Travell, USA, Robin Mackenzie, New Zealand and Freddie Kaltenborn, Norway. After two years observing physicians, osteopathic physicians and physiotherapists I became fairly competent at understanding the indications, contraindications and techniques of manipulating the spinal joints.

Impressed by the efficacy of manipulation on some cases of joint dysfunction in the cervical, thoracic and lumbar spines I offered a report on these cases. I thought 1967 was an appropriate year to acknowledge the centenary of Sir James Paget's lecture on bonesetting.[22] It amazed me that the medical profession had generally shown so little interest in the subject. For it was in 1867 that Paget had advised physicians, "Learn then to imitate what is good and avoid what is bad in the practice of bonesetters...." Few doctors followed his advice.

Lancet rejected my manuscript but wrote me such a polite letter, (as I believe they usually do), that I felt quite pleased to receive it. The Canadian Medical Association Journal sent a more blunt rejection. I later learned from an ex-editor that that journal would not touch any article on the subject. Curiously, the Medical Journal of Australia appeared quite happy to publish my first study, "Spinal manipulation in medical practice. A century of Ignorance," 1968, some 15 years after graduation.[201]

I was concerned that I might injure someone. Dr. Bill Gibson, the physician and neurophysiologist under whom I had worked, advised me to be extra careful and mentioned the articles in the Journal of the American Medical Association concerning injury following spinal manipulation, particularly neck manipulation.[202,203] I therefore determined to discover how frequently spinal manipulation caused injury, recording any prior injuries by any practitioner on 676 consecutive patients who I examined in my practice between May 15, 1966 and May 15, 1969. Three hundred and sixty-six patients were part of my regular practice while 310 were referred to me by other physicians. One hundred and seventy-two of the patients had visited a chiropractor at some time during their lives. Twelve out of the 172 patients had received some sort of injury of which four were serious.[23] In May 1966, a 31-year-old mechanic presenting to me with low back pain had visited a chiropractor two years previously. He stated that he lay on a table and the chiropractor stood on a high stool and jumped onto his back with both knees. He suffered severe pain following this incident and was unable to work for two weeks. (I should add I have never heard another similar story).

In July 1967, an 82 year-old retired pharmacist complained of low back pain for 12 months and right leg numbness for two months. X-rays of his lumbar spine August 1966 were normal. In June and July 1967 a chiropractor treated him by direct pressure to his lumbar spine as he lay prone. This tough old British Columbia pioneer said, "he was pretty rough on me." His leg numbness increased. Examination July 1967 showed questionable numbness to pin-prick on the outside of the right leg and foot. Straight leg raising of the right leg was limited to 60 degrees. Remaining neurological examination was normal. Lumbar spine x-rays disclosed wedging of the body of the third lumbar vertebra with compression on its right anterolateral aspect. I suspect, wrote the radiologist, "this injury to be comparatively recent in origin." The back pain was finally shown to be due to secondary prostatic carcinoma. It improved partly with estrogen therapy.

In April 1968, a middle-aged woman experiencing anterior chest pain at the 5th left costochondral junction and suffering from rheumatoid arthritis was treated some 40 times by a chiropractor who pressed directly upon her thoracic spine. Her mother had had a similar pain some years previously and three months later "was all skin and bones." Her daughter's natural deep seated fear of cancer explained her pain which was likely also aggravated by the excessive chiropractic treatment.

In November 1968 a 70 year-old man was hospitalized with upper back pain, mid-sternal pain, feet numbness and difficulty urinating for one week. A chiropractor had manipulated his thoracic spine. Following his third treatment the patient developed anesthesia below the level of the ninth thoracic vertebra and leg weakness. Examination confirmed anesthesia below T9. There were no reflex abnormalities. Hemoglobin 12.4 g/100 ml. Leucocyte count 15,200; neutrophils 55, eosinophils 3, staff cells 4, metamyelocytes 1, lymphocytes 17, monocytes 4, plasma cells 8, pro-plasma cells 8. ESR 38, alkaline phosphatase 88, acid phosphatase, 5.2 IU. Bone marrow examination confirmed the diagnosis of multiple myeloma. X-rays disclosed osteolytic metastatic deposits in the anterior part of the skull. A myelogram suggested an incomplete block at T8.

The patient quickly became paraplegic and died of broncho-pneumonia within a month. Autopsy revealed his spinal cord compressed by a soft tissue mass of plasmocytoma, a type of cancer.

I saw no patients with vertebral artery dysfunction following manipulation. However, such cases would likely be referred to a neurologist.[202]

Four patients treated by manipulation had no indication for it, for example in a 34 year-old man suffering from progressive loss of sight due to Eales disease where bleeding occurs in the retina of the eye. The chiropractor massaged the patient's facial muscles for three months before the patient realized he was being duped.

Damage from spinal manipulation can occur when the symptoms are not due to joint dysfunction, when the cause of the problem is unknown or when the techniques are incorrectly or too forcefully applied. Damage may also occur when logical medical assessment and treatment are delayed while useless treatment is being persisted with. Chiropractors suffer from narrow vision.

I do not believe any of the patients sued the particular chiropractor or notified chiropractic authorities. Thus most chiropractors are unaware of the frequency of injury.

One Australian chiropractor reviewing vascular injury following neck manipulation claimed that they injure only one in ten million patients.[204] The 1971 study suggests such claim to be false.[23] However, chiropractors have earned some patients' respect due to their use of manipulation, a skill doctors generally have failed to learn.[22] I suspect chiropractors are most grateful to the medical profession for such omission. Chiropractic training is improving, and I know two teachers who are trying hard to improve standards. Nevertheless, patients are still being seriously injured.[27,205]

As I continued further studies on spinal manipulation,[206] I began to wonder how many other Canadian GPs had completed research. Discussing the matter with Dr. Donald Williams, Associate Dean of Medicine at the University of British Columbia in 1967, I found him unaware of any research done by any GP in Canada. Looking at me quite kindly he remarked,

"It's a pity you are not doing your research at the university. We could get it published for you then. You will never get published on your own."

However, his comment stimulated me to find what research GPs had done in Canada. I wrote to appropriate journals asking readers to notify me of any. During the next four years I completed four articles on the subject.[207-210] I came across Dr. Ian McWhinney's extensive clinical research which he began while in the UK, writing on a wide variety of topics such as ischemic heart disease, brucellosis, thyroiditis, depression, cancer diagnosis, and the status and need for the general practitioner. In 1969 he wrote,[211]

"The success of the scientific revolution in medicine has changed the pattern of disease, increased the demand for medical care, and fragmented the profession into specialties. The crux of our present dilemma is the inability of a fragmented profession to satisfy the needs of a people whose health problems are multiple and chronic."

Besides McWhinney I found some 21 Canadian general practitioners performing research on a wide variety of topics in the 1950-1970 period. [201,212-231]

Probably I failed to find three or four others.

I noted their age, size of their community, type of practice, medical school and length of post graduate study. The results are summarised at the end of the chapter in Table 1. I record only their first study. Interested parties can refer to their other work in references quoted in the 1974 article.[210]

It takes time to understand general practice. The average age of the researchers on performing their first study was 40.6 years. Only four researchers practised in Canada's largest cities - Montreal, Toronto, Edmonton and Vancouver. Most practised in smaller centres. Malyska worked in Deloraine, Manitoba, population 1,000, Scott in Loon Lake, Saskatchewan, population 800 and McAnulty, Oyama, Winfield, B.C. population 2,000. Three graduated from Edinburgh and five from Toronto. Eight were solo practitioners. It takes dedication to do research in a small population. Libraries are far distant while encouragement is lacking. Small town practitioners have additional responsibilities.

Amoebic dysentery is associated with tropical countries but Frank Scott discovered an epidemic in Loon Lake,[228] McAnulty[222] noted the menace of raw or partially treated sewage in lagoons, and became unpopular with certain politicians. Malyska[225] investigated the value of autohypnosis in antenatal patients, noting the ease of later delivery and the low rate of caesarean section. All three physicians practised in small towns.

GP/family doctors treat about 50 percent of the nation's sick but contribute less than 1 percent to the medical literature. Generally speaking they find it difficult to obtain publication, but, they must try to record their unique observations. Incidentally, Australian practitioners have researched more.[207] Today, research is being carried out in University departments of family practice, but the <u>Canadian Family Physician</u> records few studies by those practising in regular communities. I expect that non-university practitioners also reported their observations in the United States, in the UK and elsewhere.

While completing these studies I was asked to lead the local hospital's education program for medical student training.

18

TEACHING STUDENTS IN THE COMMUNITY

One century ago the noted American educator, Abraham Flexner, undertook to evaluate and improve the state of medical education in North America. In the teaching schools of the time he found,[232]

"A school that began in October would graduate a class the next spring....the student registered in the office of a physician he never saw.

He no longer read his master's books, submitted to his quizzing, or rode with him the countryside in the <u>enjoyment of valuable bedside opportunities</u>. (my underlining). All the training that a young doctor got before beginning his practice had to be procured within the medical school. The school was no longer a supplement, it was everything."

Flexner found deficiencies in even the more select schools. For example, some practitioners had used the stethoscope for over 30 years before it was mentioned in the Harvard medical school catalogue.[232] Flexner believed (as can be seen from the earlier quote) that apprenticeship still had its place in student education.

However, following his report many schools and apprenticeships were abolished and students instructed by University hospital teachers.

Generally, such changes were beneficial, but, as students became taught upon rarer hospitalized cases in teaching hospitals they were less exposed to patients with commoner problems in the community and became separated from the community.

Increased scientific knowledge led to increasing specialization with its rewards, prestige and intellectual satisfaction, but also, increased fragmentation of care. To aim for more reality-based education among students and to improve communication between university and the community Dean Bardeen initiated a preceptorship program at the University of Wisconsin where students became assigned to physicians in regular practice. In 1928 he reported in the Journal of the <u>American Medical Association,</u>[233]

"Fundamental training in the science can only be well-given at the universities. The art, however, cannot be well-taught if the teachers of science at the university do not work in cooperation with and have the hearty cooperation of those who are actually practising medicine as an art."

Forty-four years later Sivertson and Stone found the Wisconsin program still flourishing.[234] Other centres such as Western Reserve in 1952, along with Illinois, Kansas, Duke, Rochester, Harvard, Pennsylvania and Washington State began various family practice-oriented teaching programs. In 1974 Washington combined with Montana, Idaho and Alaska to form a four State teaching block using community physicians to teach medical students in outlying areas.[235]

Various reports such as the Millis commission.[236] The Folsom commission[237] and the Willard report[238] stimulated the development of these programs, revealing that most Americans wanted a personal physician, broadly and relevantly trained, able to provide urgent, comprehensive and continuing medical care to families in the community. [236-238]

In 1970, the University of British Columbia, Canada, started an educational experiment in which final year medical students would be attached to a community hospital during a three month elective program.

Students had alternative opportunities during their elective such as working in the emergency department at the Vancouver General

Hospital or in the family practice teaching unit in Vancouver or doing three months in any other discipline.

In 1970, 35 students out of a class of 60 chose a community hospital program. By 1974 that program attracted 58 students out of a class of 75. Meanwhile four students attended the family practice teaching unit in 1970, dropping to none in 1974. By then 17 communities had become involved.

In 1971, two local physicians, the late Dr. Arnold Emery and Dr. Michael Livingston were asked by the Richmond hospital to take charge of the teaching program at the hospital. During that year six students participated. After a few months experience we thought it could prove valuable to obtain the students' opinion of Richmond hospital's teaching program. So we gave six consecutive students a simple questionnaire to base their reports upon.[239] We stressed to the students their reports, limited to 250 words, would be anonymous and unedited. They would be co-authors of any published account.

Richmond was a growing Vancouver suburb whose population in 1971 was 66,000. The community hospital of 151 beds also attracted patients from neighbouring communities. There were 28 family doctors and 26 specialists on active staff and 99 other physicians with visiting privileges. We divided students' time between medicine, surgery, obstetrics, pediatrics and the emergency department. Students spent three afternoons a week in the offices of family physicians and two afternoons with a specialist of their choice. After six weeks students changed to different family physicians and specialists.

About a quarter of the family physicians and a few specialists did not wish to have students in their offices. Specialists provided about 50 percent of the teaching, family doctors 45 percent and other personnel five percent. Students worked every second or third night and every second or third week-end.

Here are the questions and the complete unedited replies of two students, also short quotations from the four other students.[239]

QUESTIONS:

1. List your primary objectives in pursuing the Elective Program. Did you achieve them?

2. Describe your impressions of family medicine as regards:
(a) Community hospital setting
(b) Family doctor's office practice
(c) Specialist practice
(d) Learning experiences in Emergency
3. Make general comments, criticisms and recommendations re clerkship elective program, compare with previous teaching experiences re standards, interest, various specialties, etc.
4. Would you be more inclined to enter family practice on the basis of this experience?

Replies - Student 1
1. Objectives
(a). Realistic exposure to, and practice in, family medicine.
(b). Practical experience in the routine procedures.
(c). To investigate the organization and workings of a smaller community hospital.
(d). An informal exposure to medical economics.
These four objectives have been satisfactorily achieved.
2. Impressions of family medicine
a). The community-based hospital which cares for the health needs of people in a given geographic area, which is self-contained, which is accessible to family doctors, and which is of fewer than 500 beds, appears to be an excellent form of health care
(b). G.P. office practice exposure was very worth-while from two points of view:
i. Method and content of a family doctor's practice.

ii. Variety of methods for handling similar problems in different practices.

(c). Specialist practice: Highlight of this aspect was the willingness of most specialists to teach informally. ENT, dermatology, O & G, and orthopedic office exposure was valuable. Of special note was the opportunity to help with several cardiac arrests.

(d) Emergency Department learning experiences were innumerable. Some examples i. I have become proficient in the suturing of most minor lacerations and reduction of minor fractures. ii. I have had opportunity to handle several drug overdoses, several car accidents, cardiac arrests. iii. Emergency care and investigation of a coronary case. iv. The handling of acute violent psychosis.

Comments - (a). The clerkship elective program is basically a very good idea. Time in family medicine should be a core part of every medical student's training, especially when most internships emphasize specialty practice. I have been generally satisfied with my time at R.G.H. There have been only a few features that have marred the experience:

1. Not being called for a number of deliveries despite having previously requested nursing staff to notify me.

2. O.R. staff becoming impatient with slowness of externes in operating, closing an incision, etc.

3. The constant worry by the nursing staff about scheduling their coffee and lunch breaks (unions!) 4. Having to call a doctor about Emergency Department patients, no matter how small the problem.

The teaching is just as good as that at the Vancouver General Hospital although less formalized. An advantage is that teaching is available when one asks for it. It is not forced on a student or mercilessly scheduled. The friendly atmosphere is notable. The lack of obligation to do "scut-work" is a very welcome aspect of the elective.

The opportunity to look after cases varied greatly. Some physicians allowed virtually complete control whereas others allowed none. A directive to the nursing staff explaining the function of the externes would be advisable.

I found internal medicine the most interesting specialty field while at Richmond General Hospital.

Specific negative highlights:

1. Dr. X has considerable talent at producing surgical morbidity.

2. Dr. Y is very thorough and a good example to Dr. Z who treats pneumonia over the phone.

3. Do Lab and X-ray truly run the hospital? People get sick on weekends!

4. I am definitely more inclined to do family practice after this R.G.H. experience. I certainly hope R.G.H. continues its externe program.

Replies - Student 2

1. The community hospital offered:

(a) An exposure to general practice.

(b) An escape from the large referral hospital where "scut-work" is frequently demanded in the name of education and dissatisfaction is normal.

2. Impressions:

(a) Community hospital - bright pleasant and busy.

A high standard of medicine. A typical day might include:

Morning - medical rounds, minor to major surgery (to operate or assist), an autopsy with the pathologist, reading films with the radiologist, a delivery any time (over 60 patients delivered by me) Afternoon - in an office or on the wards.

Evening - the library, maternity unit, intensive care unit, emergency - the latter a steady stream of lacerations, head injuries, fractures, chest and abdominal problems, drug overdoses, pediatric and psychiatric problems, many treated by me, all evaluated first hand.

An inexhaustible variety of clinical material, an eager and knowledgeable group of physicians to guide and teach.

(b) Office practice - solo, partnership, group, high volume, low volume, how to make and lose money, superb medicine, adequate medicine. General practice takes intuition and a

thick skin. Specialists are slick, make more accurate
diagnoses and focus more on diseases than people.
All offer something, all candid without exception.
I enjoyed them all. An absolutely necessary exposure to
the non-acute care of the public.

3. The experience is valuable. The student sees office practice
which is reality-based, not idealistic and subsidized. He is listened
to, expected to take responsibility, to learn proper use of limited
diagnostic facilities and to enjoy himself. It works if he works. It should
be continued.

4. Yes. This experience encourages me to enter family practice.

Student 3 commented that "suddenly medicine became alive....
There is ample opportunity to see patients without standing in line
behind residents."

"In a family doctor's office practice one sees bread and butter
medicine, which is not experienced in a hospital environment, and the
entire sequence of events in the health care system, e.g. antenatal visit,
case room experience, postnatal visit.

Specialties such as ENT and dermatology can only be learned in
the office since only the rare and complicated cases reach hospital."

Student 4 observed that "the program complemented and made
more meaningful university teaching."

Student 5 wrote that "the office experience was excellent. I saw
many minor conditions never seen in major centres and also some
uncommon diseases, e.g. acute gout, sub acute combined degeneration,
pityriasis rosea and orchitis. Dr. X gave a convincing demonstration
of manipulation. I observed counselling with Dr. Y. Dr. Z does a lot of
pediatrics." He added "clinical professors have more to say but here I
could observe and read as I wished."

Student 6 stressed the value of the emergency department and the
opportunity to follow patients. "The great advantage here as contrasted
to Emergency rotations elsewhere is the chance to follow the case

in the O.R., on the wards, and not infrequently in the doctor's own office." "Office practice as seen so far calls for a lot of skin, eye, ENT and orthopedics, which are not covered enough in medical school, but three months here makes up a great part of the deficit."

Student 7

He approached his learning experience with some bias. As he noted in his full report, he had received the impression from his University teachers that, "The GP is nothing, knows nothing, is seldom involved, and is only a tool to channel patients to the appropriate specialist." He continued "I must say the most valuable experience, in fact the only opportunity during the four years training in U.B.C. medical school, is to be able to see the GPs in actual practice in the afternoons. There one can see the variation of method and content of practice between the doctors, and can also compare a group practice with a solo practice. Most of the GPs I met in Richmond are more capable than I expected and did a good job in explaining their practice, sometimes even the financial side of it."

Student 8

"It is Interesting to see how the GP screens out patients and deals with functional and organic problems, whereas the specialist has the advantage (?) of dealing with definable organic problems. It is the family doctor who can keep things in perspective for the patient, e.g. specialist advises surgery but patient turns to GP for interpretation and support. The family doctor is more personable – and so he should be. The specialist sees the patient on only one or two occasions and obviously will not develop the same relationship."

Some educators might question the quality of student teaching in the community and students' ability to judge that quality, because some previous studies have noted deficiencies among community doctors. [241,242]

(1) However student 1 was able to note both
 positive and negative aspects of the teaching (my underlining)
(2) All students approved the opportunity for
 direct patient contact.

"Without standing in line behind residents," as student 3 remarked.

(3) They appreciated learning basic skills and following patients' progress.

(4) They appreciated seeing common problems not seen in the medical school setting. Student 5.

(5) They valued delivering under supervision an average of 35 babies each, an experience hard to obtain in most medical schools.

(6) Most approved exposure to the social aspect of medicine, for many medical students are "socially ignorant." [243]

(7) The first eight students and four later ones provided consistent replies. They wished to leave the school setting and "go out and do something." [244]

(8) They valued visiting both GPs and specialists in their offices and seeing office orthopedics, dermatology, O & G and ENT.

(9) Student 2 summarized the office experience thus, All offer something, all candid without exception. I enjoyed them all. An absolutely necessary exposure to the non-acute care of the public. (my underlining.)

(10) Student 1 summarized the whole experience,

"The clerkship elective program is basically a very good idea. Time in family medicine should be a core part of every medical student's training, especially when most internships emphasize specialty practice." (my underlining.)

Of interest, the first two students to enter the program later returned to Richmond to enter family practice.

Further comment

1. The program is simple and inexpensive. The patients, doctors and buildings are all present. Teachers received no remuneration.

2. All medical students responded positively to the Richmond training program. As time passed, the word "got around" and we received increasing inquiries about our program from Canada and beyond. Lion's Gate hospital in North Vancouver also proved most

popular, as did others. "Natural selection" occurred. Students learned from other students of those hospitals offering better programs and applied to work there.

3. While some university teachers question the calibre of teaching, [241-242] others do not. Sedal from Australia suggested GPs take part in teaching[245] while Balint urged they should leave their pupil position and rise to the challenge of teaching.[246] Is it reasonable for students to spend all their educational years at the university isolated from the community and taught by teachers who have never experienced general practice themselves?[159]

4. Do family practice teaching units at university hospitals provide the breadth of clinical experiences that can be achieved in the community setting? Lloyd [247] from the Montreal General Hospital pointed out some of the barriers such as artificial settings, unrealistic hours and the impossibility of continuous relationships.

5. Have other community hospital teaching programs proved successful? By 1975 the program at Wisconsin had continued for 47 years.[233,234] Sivertson and Stone noting challenges to their program sent out questionnaires to 468 students of the classes of 1934, 1944, 1959, 1964, 1968 and 1970. Of those replying, 218 considered the program should remain as a requirement, 69 felt it should be elective and only one advocated its abandonment. At the time of their paper Wisconsin had only one requirement during the students' fourth year, namely the preceptorship program.[234]

6. Besides benefiting students with reality-based education the medical and paramedical staff benefited from having inquiring students present, in effect encouraging their continuing education.

7. Reaching time scheduling at the medical school is always at a premium among competing disciplines. When family practice teachers attempted to get a foothold in medical schools they soon experienced opposition. As Dr. Gayle Stephens put it in his work, The Intellectual Basis of Family Practice. [248]

"The medical education establishment has proved to be a tough opponent, with weapons we never dreamed of. Not only has academia turned out to be less liberal than we had supposed, but sometimes cranky and ill-tempered...."

Interestingly, at Richmond, we found that students staying three months could obtain a really valuable experience. It took some students three weeks to find their feet and a similar time for the staff to trust their individual ability and judgment.

Suddenly, without warning, the program was cut to eight weeks, severely restricting its benefits. Soon, the program was cut further. Apparently, no one at the university fought hard enough for its continuance. We suspect that its very success had encouraged opposition by some teachers.

As students stayed for shorter periods, relationship between them and the medical staff failed to develop, inevitably weakening the program and reducing the enthusiasm that had developed in the local physician community.

Others' more recent observations

In 1999 Leone-Perkins et al. from Philadelphia[251] found that overall 594 third-year students taking four week rotations at community and residency-based sites rated their experience favourably. From our experience in Richmond we are surprised that a four week program was satisfactory, and suggest they try a longer program[239,240,244]

In the UK the General Medical Council recommended more community-based teaching in a directive published in 1993.[252] In 2002 Drs Coleman and Murray[253] described how patients viewed teaching when pairs or small groups of students were instructed by general practitioners in the patients' homes or doctors' offices in North London. Patients were recruited for this experience and were told it could involve a two hour visit and that they would not be attending for routine medical care.

Most patients approved of the experience. They felt that broadening students' education in the community should lead to improved service later in communities. Some felt it was an opportunity to repay the system, one patient stating, " I feel sort of slightly as if I'm giving a bit back, because I've had a lot out of the health service." Patients unable to work due to chronic illness found being involved in teaching gave them pleasure and a sense of worth. Some felt less isolated and others appreciated being so thoroughly examined.[253]

A minority feared embarrassment. One patient constantly going to doctors or to the hospital, wanted to "get away from it all." Of course patients volunteered to enter the program.

In an earlier article[254] Dr. Murray had reviewed the challenges and rewards to medical students of community-based teaching by general practitioners. Murray noted that much of their research could be applied internationally.

In the US, Dr. Ferenchick et al [255] in 2002 reviewed 22 articles on community-based teaching, concluding that both students and teachers benefited from the experience. Students benefitted particularly from learning to recognise disease patterns, managing chronic illness and psychosocial problems when compared to their other traditional clerkship rotations.

Other recent articles I have searched do not add significantly to the subject.

To summarize, some 30 years after our experience in Richmond, Canada, and 75 years after Dean Bardeen's program at Wisconsin, the benefits of teaching medical students in the community are being slowly realized. In view of our experience in Richmond,[239,240] I strongly urge a 10-12 week program for all students, preferably at the end of their 3rd academic year when they have received basic grounding.

Three months training at the community level seem small indeed compared to four years at the university. We should remember Dr. Kerr White et al. [256] had previously reported that only a small fraction of patients require treatment at a university hospital.

It is particularly important that students considering specialty training first experience training in the community, for this will likely prove to be their only such experience.

If community-based teaching programs are to succeed,

1. The central director must believe in the program.
2. Preceptors must be adequately trained and respond to students' needs.
3. Students must work.
4. Local physicians, the community and the university

must communicate fully and be equal partners.

Finally, by encouraging an adequate training program in the community the medical profession will be following the wishes of the community.[240-255]

In British Columbia more training in the community is being encouraged at programs in Prince George and Victoria during 2005.

19

ALTERNATIVE MEDICINE

We have seen how opportunities for research may occur when patients visit family doctors. In chapter 6, I missed an opportunity by failing to listen sufficiently to one patient who might have told me something of the origins of manipulative treatment in his native African country.

In February 1984 another opportunity arose when three new patients who had attended alternative practitioners consulted me about their backs on the same day. Here are their stories.

In reporting these anecdotal accounts one relies in part upon the accuracy of the patients' tales. Generally, medical editors disapprove of anecdotal reports, but such reports may provide valid information not learned in other ways.[257]

BRIEF CASE REPORTS

Patient referred by Dr. Peter Chang M.D.

An unemployed 20-year-old North American Chinese woman YMCA exercise teacher developed sudden low back pain in June 1983, but continued dancing.

Her family doctor reassured her, advised rest and medication without effect. She was referred to a rheumatologist who diagnosed a short right leg and recommended raising her right heel. Her pain worsened. A physiotherapist at a sports medicine clinic gave her 16 electrical treatments but apparently no education. No change. Then she turned to alternative healers, visiting three different chiropractors during the next few months who gave differing opinions. A full body x-ray from one apparently "revealed": a high right pelvis, a high right ear, a low right shoulder, a displaced second cervical vertebra, a displaced thoracic vertebra, a sacrum twisted to the left, left pelvis twisted to the front and a short right leg.

Currently she was attending a chiropractor who "just touches your neck, making a specially delicate adjustment," so delicate that the patient would not allow me to examine her neck for fear I might disturb it.

Therefore, I spent time explaining the multiple reasons for pain, - injury, posture, tension, past and family experience; and taught her balanced relaxation exercises she could do at home to help her own recovery. She did not return.

Patient referred by Dr. Don Stewart M.D.

A 56 year-old real estate agent stated she was injured in her fourth (rather minor) motor vehicle accident 4 1/2 months previously and still experienced severe low and mid-back pain. She had consulted her family doctor who agreed with her visiting a chiropractor. After three months of little benefit, her doctor suggested a physiotherapist who seemed more helpful, but he went on holiday and she felt worse under his replacement. A podiatrist said her feet were in terrible shape and her back would never improve until her feet were right. Then the patient saw a reflexologist. Essentially, her condition was unchanged.

Examination revealed minimal objective findings, some pain following hyperextension of the lumbar spine. She cried profusely during her visit and seemed primarily to be suffering from anxiety-tension-depression.

I explained the natural course of her condition to her and gave a simple daily exercise program stressing flexion exercises, walking, and attending fewer therapists.

The guitarist

A young guitarist had experienced low back pain for two weeks aggravated by sitting and bending forward and backward. His straight leg raising was limited to 60 degrees on the right side. He had no neurological abnormalities, but examination showed trigger points to the right of his 5th lumbar vertebra and in his right gluteus medius (buttock) muscle.

While I discussed with him the natural history of his condition, taught him three basic back exercises he could do daily, encouraged daily walking and used one manipulation to the right of his 5th lumbar vertebra, he told me of a previous episode three years earlier.

He had experienced low back pain for two years and received 20 ultrasound treatments from a physiotherapist whom he stated taught him no exercise rehabilitation. Nor did the chiropractor teach him much despite adjusting his vertebrae some 70 times. Curiously, he thought the chiropractor was good.

His back was still somewhat sore while he was on a musical tour, visiting Regina, Saskatchewan, Canada. He was walking with his wife on the outskirts of the city when a large jackrabbit jumped up on the edge of the pavement and bounded along the sidewalk. "Something came back to me from my childhood and I started to chase after the jackrabbit. The rabbit turned sharply right, I tried to turn also, but slipped on the ground, landing on my back. I got up and the pain had gone."

The jackrabbit adjustment had succeeded where 20 physiotherapy visits and 70 chiropractic adjustments had failed.

All three patients were overtreated yet apparently were not

taught reasonable exercise rehabilitation they could do to help their own recovery. Their management was indeed variable. Today physiotherapists would be more inclined to teach exercises.

Despite the advances of orthodox medicine during the past century, people consult alternative practitioners increasingly. Eisenberg et al. from Harvard Medical School reported that Americans made 425 million visits to alternative health care providers in 1990, more than they visited allopathic (orthodox) primary care physicians during the same period.[258] Why?

In Alternative Medicine and Ethics, 1998, Stephen Barrett and Vimal Patel debated the value of alternative Medicine.[259,260]

Barrett, a board member of the National Council Against Health Fraud, studied alternative medicine for years and stated that "Alternative" medicine has at least one of the following characteristics:

1. Its rationale or underlying theory has no scientific basis.

2. It has not been demonstrated safe and effective by well-designed studies.

3. It is deceptively promoted.

4. Its practitioners are not qualified to make appropriate diagnoses.

"Alternative" practitioners claim they promote general health and are cost-effective against chronic illness. However there is no published evidence that they persuade patients to adopt a more healthy lifestyle than do mainstream physicians.

Patel acknowledged the successes of modern medicine in communicable diseases, emergency medicine and surgically treatable structural abnormalities. However, he believed the health care industry had focused its energies on "disease care" rather than health care. He pointed out that in overcrowded and polluted Shanghai, life expectancy exceeded that of New York City and the cost for health care was far less.[260]

Patel emphasized the chronic disease crisis in the US, and a current health care system which was too technological and impersonal. He claimed that a Cartesian/Newtonian biomedical model guided modern medicine and nearly ignored the role of mind and spirit in illness.

Others have discussed various facets of alternative medicine.[261-263]

Why have alternative healers become so popular? I suggest some of the following reasons:

1. They may appeal to people from a different culture who are comfortable with a particular form of therapy such as acupuncture.

2. They may appeal to people who yearn for more natural living and question medicine's emphasis upon drugs and technology.

3. Patients may have experienced little success or reasonable concern from a mainstream physician and try a different remedy recommended by a friend.

4. Most of us have experienced visiting a healer, mainstream or alternative and feeling better following that visit. Michael Balint[264] emphasized that the doctor himself is very powerful medicine. Whoever the healer is receives reasonable credit for that effect.

5. Most illnesses are self-limiting. The practitioner receives undeserved credit for the cure.

6. Doctors have ignored certain useful techniques available to them if they wish to study beyond their initial training. For example, we noted earlier how James Paget over a century ago advised doctors to "imitate what is good...in the practise of bonesetters."[22] He was ignored and osteopaths and later chiropractors filled the void.

7. Alternative healers treat mostly an ambulant population. Modern medicine may involve expensive technology, multiple referrals and hospitalization.

8. Alternative healers concentrate upon providing hope.

9. Confusion and suspicion exists about science. Drugs or investigations may help or may cause side-effects.

10. The Media, quite happy to criticise orthodox medicine, tends to promote the unorthodox and newsworthy.

11. Ignorance. Few people are aware of the lack of standards and sometimes outright deceptions of some alternative healers. One example should suffice.

A young man just returned from a business trip in Japan consulted me about his sore lower back. He related the following tale.

His host had noticed him struggling to rise from the conference table and recommended the young man consult an acupuncturist he knew. The patient hobbled into the one-room office and eased himself into a chair. There were two treatment tables in the room separated by a flimsy screen. A patient lay on each table.

Having nothing better to do the young man watched the acupuncturist at work. To his horror he saw the acupuncturist take the needles out of one patient's body and insert them directly into the other. There was no attempt at sterilising the needles or even wiping any blood off them.

The young man struggled to his feet. "I got out of there as fast as I could," he exclaimed. He realised the possibility of transferring infection. AIDS or hepatitis C could be transferred in this way.

I do not wish to imply that other acupuncturists practise in this manner. However, patients should ask practitioners about their sterilisation methods. Individual packaged sterilised needles are available.

Patients should also realise that herbs widely touted as being natural and safe may cause serious side-effects, for example, the foxglove leaf.[154-156] Herbs may also conflict with prescribed medication, a point to remember.[262]

12. The obsession with health in our society noted by Thomas Lewis in Medusa and the Snail.[265]

13. The decline of the generalist in medicine, (discussed in the previous chapter) not only of the general practitioner but also of the general internist. People want someone reasonably able, available and amiable, who will provide continuing care and whom they can trust with their health problems. If the medical profession does not provide, people will search beyond it.

14. Finally, alternative healers usually have limited treatment options. So they concentrate upon the most important. They listen to, touch and take time to convince patients.

Greenhalgh and Hurwitz provide a simple example of a patient who consulted his general practitioner over three years for advice to help him quit smoking. His GP tried all the known methods without success. The patient then visited a complementary (alternative) practitioner who "advised him to draw up a legal contract with himself.

This was to state the date on which he intended to quit, and was to be signed and witnessed. From that date he never smoked again."[266]

Inadvertently, science may block physicians communicating with their patients. As Norman Cousins commented,[267]

"Every time you go to a referral or to a diagnostic machine, you are increasing the distance between yourself and the doctor who is such a powerful ingredient in helping set you right."

Could alternative healers be showing the medical profession the path to more effective healing - closer contact and communication with patients?

Any practitioner who listens, encourages balanced exercise and nutrition, a purpose for living and avoids over-medicating will help many patients.

We should not forget that alternative medicine has as long a tradition as emperico-rational medicine, for in ancient Egypt magical and religious and rational medicine ran side by side.[268] Besides reviewing some facets of alternative medicine, this chapter provides an example of simple clinical research, reporting four cases with certain similarities, then searching the literature widely and offering suggestions based upon the patients, study and experience. A doctor's office and patients continue to offer opportunities to the persistent observer.

The tale is evidence.

20

A NEW WHIPLASH DISCOVERY

Whiplash is not an injury, it is a whip lash, a whipping movement. The whiplash mystery began with its name and lack of definition. Indeed, the whiplash problem even started before the popularity of the modern car. In 1971, Toronto orthopedic surgeon Ian Macnab noted that acceleration extension forces (whipping forces) to the cervical spine were observed among World War I pilots catapulted abruptly from warships. Some pilots crashed into the sea likely due to disorientation or blackouts following extreme rapid neck movement.[269] The problem was solved by raising the level of the pilot's seat to reduce neck extension.

Macnab attributed the term "whiplash" to another orthopedic surgeon, Harold Crowe, who referred to the whiplike motion of the head in some car accidents at a 1928 meeting of orthopedic surgeons in San Francisco.[270] Crowe came to regret his use of the term which stimulated people's imagination and became hugely popular in America. In 1945 the term entered a major journal when A.G. Davis reported 134 cases of cervical spine injury in the <u>Journal of the</u>

American Medical Association.[271] He noted that the great majority of cases among ambulant patients were in the nature of a "whip lash," and considered that whiplash occurred most frequently in head-on collisions when hyperflexion of the head was followed by extension. Interestingly, most ambulant patients recovered within days.

Eight years later neurosurgeons Gay and Abbott reported a small series of 50 patients with "common whiplash injuries of the neck," also in the JAMA.[272] In contrast to Davis's observations they found that 90 percent of patients were occupants in motor vehicles struck from behind. Curiously, the authors claimed that their patients' heads also bent forward acutely after impact, (despite the impact being opposite to Davis's patients!) When a car is struck forcefully from behind it is surely reasonable for the occupant's unsupported head to first bend backwards, not forwards. The whiplash mystery deepened.

Gay and Abbott also claimed that the initial movement was sometimes followed by "several less violent oscillations of the neck in alternating flexion and extension." A somewhat fanciful notion. Much investigation and debate on the mechanics of "whiplash injury" followed.[273,30,274]

Gay and Abbott reported symptoms following the accident such as bewilderment, head and neck pain, and limb paresthesiae, but apparently did not inquire into any pre-existing symptoms. They described some cars being driven ahead "several hundred feet" by the impact. They discussed the development of a most distressing psychoneurotic reaction in 52 percent of patients.

Articles continued to flow from the JAMA including those by Gotten (1956),[275] Schutt and Dohan (1968),[276] and Farbmann (1973).[39] Farbmann eschewed the dramatic diagnosis of "whiplash injury," commenting that many conditions were lumped together under that heading and limited his study to 136 patients with "simple, uncomplicated musculoligamentous sprain, the most common of all neck injuries." At last we have a clear description.

One day during 1992 I was searching through the whiplash literature at the excellent British Columbia Medical Library when I made a simple discovery. Anyone researching whiplash thoroughly could have made it.

But apparently no one had.

When a new medical syndrome is described in a major journal on one side of the Atlantic it invariably surfaces in a major journal on the other side within three years. However, such surfacing did not occur in the whiplash mystery. I searched <u>Lancet</u>, the <u>British Medical Journal</u> and the British edition of the <u>Journal of Bone and Joint Surgery</u> from 1953 to 1983. There was no report of whiplash injury or neck sprain among British patients during those years. Indeed, it was not until 1983 that Norris and Watt [277] described the prognosis of neck injuries after rear-end collisions in 61 patients presenting to the accident department of the Bristol Royal Infirmary over a 32-month period.

Three years later the <u>British Medical Journal</u> published Deans et al's study on the incidence and duration of neck pain in a sample of 137 traceable patients who had attended a Belfast hospital in Northern Ireland following a motor vehicle collision. [278]

Why the 30-year reporting gap between North American and British patients? Unbelievable.

Some readers might consider that British editors refused articles on the subject, but such refusal is unlikely to occur in a number of journals. To me the only reasonable explanation for the reporting gap was that British patients were not experiencing enough symptoms following neck sprains after motor vehicle collisions to draw the attention of researchers.

In particular, London, a huge city packed with taxis and other motor vehicles must have witnessed numerous rear-end collisions between 1953 and 1983. London contained many medical schools where traffic accident victims were treated in casualty departments and whose teaching staff would have been only too delighted to explore a new syndrome.

But they did not.

In effect, British patients had not copied North American ones. One must wonder over the reasons for the difference. But one thing is surely likely: the reasons would be social rather than mechanical. For example, some might speculate that the quantity and input of lawyers in America could be one factor.

I sent a letter to <u>Lancet</u> on the observation and then a short article to the editor of the Journal of the Royal Society of Medicine. Usually as a researcher, one has to wait months before hearing about the fate of an article; but, to my surprise, within five weeks I received a friendly reply from the editor, accepting the article, "Whiplash injury and peer-copying." It was a relief to find that an editor of a classic journal had considered the observations worth publishing.[279] I also mentioned the mysterious gap in two other articles,[280,281] hoping someone would pick up the concept of peer copying from one of the three reports. Actually six years passed before rheumatologist Robert Ferrari mentioned some of my work in The Whiplash Encyclopedia: The Facts and Myths of Whiplash in 1999,[282] and a psychiatrist, Andrew Malleson, picked up on peer copying from these articles in his critical work Whiplash and Other Useful Illnesses in 2002.[283]

Writing, as any author knows, is hard, time-consuming and often lonely work. It is not easy to obtain publication, particularly if one is just a regular practitioner or produces observations not held by most physicians or peer reviewers. Such a pattern is too common. We will consider an example later, but first, let us note examples of peer copying, not by patients but by physicians.

In 1974, Hohl,[284] an orthopedic surgeon from Beverly Hills, California, reported a poor prognosis in patients with whiplash injuries. Five years following their accidents Hohl described 43 percent of 146 patients still experiencing significant symptoms. Other authors then "peer copied" Hohl's figures.[277,278,285-287] However, none of them mentioned the vital fact that Hohl followed up merely 27 percent of his patients, a fact he mentioned in the body of his article, but failed to mention in his abstract. Such small sampling gravely affects the validity of his study, is a serious source of bias,[288] and clouds the mystery of whiplash even further. Another possible source of bias lies within his population sample. Beverly Hills could be an unusual segment of the American population.

Nevertheless, 15 years later, a British orthopedic surgeon, Porter, produced an editorial on neck sprains after car accidents for the British Medical Journal,[285] and followed Hohl's opinion closely, apparently even copying from his abstract, writing,

"...Sharp reversal of the cervical lordosis on a radiograph, restricted motion at one level on radiographs taken in flexion and extension, the use of a cervical collar for more than twelve weeks...."

The wording is very similar to that of Hohl's abstract, apart from using the British word radiographs,

"Sharp reversal of the cervical lordosis visible on roentgenograms; restricted motion at one interspace as shown by flexion - extension roentgenograms; need for a cervical collar for more than twelve weeks...."

Editorials in the British Medical Journal carry increased status.

Porter's acceptance of Hohl's opinions would have influenced practitioners, teachers, students and lawyers. Misinformation is easily perpetuated in medicine, a sorry and too frequent tale.

Meanwhile, a valid observation was ignored for years. How would you research the effects of car crashing on occupants? One obvious method would be to inquire from those participating in frequent car crashes i.e. car crashing or automobile demolition derby drivers to find what symptoms they experienced.

So thought a Toronto doctor, Philip Melville, back in the early sixties. He attended a car crashing contest outside Toronto and described the event thoroughly in a letter to the Canadian Medical Association Journal in 1963,[289] presenting his report "to bring the attention of interested physicians to bear on comparable activities and foster further scientific inquiry." "The object of the entertainment," he wrote, "is to demolish automobiles by collision... the winner being the operator of the last vehicle to move under its own power." There were 92 drivers in four heats with a final play-off.

They used ordinary road vehicles, about 10 years old with no special equipment apart from a safely belt and a white crash helmet. They used the rear-end of their cars to strike the other cars as front-ends were more vulnerable mechanically. As cars were eliminated, tail to tail collisions of "probably 50 mph or more are possible."

"The drivers are subject to a large variety of forces, from a multitude of directions, differing greatly in intensity, and both predictable and unpredictable to the busy contestants. Their heads in the large white helmets which are customary, were in particular noted to flail through a great range of movement. In spite of these factors, no significant injuries occurred."

The pit steward and the agent for the insurance company confirmed there were no injuries and that serious injury was extremely rare. When one considers that the average driver must have suffered 20 or more collisions and that many of the several thousand collisions were mechanically comparable to the rear-end accidents so common on our streets today, "the absence of cervical injury is truly remarkable compared to the apparent injuries suffered by car occupants in regular driving."

Melville hoped to draw the attention of interested physicians and "foster scientific inquiry." However his report was ignored. No one has bothered to repeat Melville's observations. Few quote his work.

Regarding the absence of injury by the participants, one might speculate that the drivers enjoyed their work of car-smashing, would be part of a group of comrades competing regularly and would "peer-copy" one another in ignoring minor symptoms, contrasting regular car occupants who would likely enter the treatment cycle and have any symptoms all-too-often reinforced by health-care providers, trying to help.

I was wrong when I wrote, "no one has bothered to repeat Melville's observations." Thanks to the searching of an enthusiastic librarian at the British Columbia Medical Library, I was introduced just yesterday to a fine article by a Toronto neurologist, Dr. Henry Berry who included among his observations a study of all 20 drivers in a 1994 car-crashing Demolition Derby in Ontario.[290] Twenty is a small sample, but Berry noted many similarities to Melville's study.[289]

The drivers averaging 29 years old had participated in Demolition Derbies for an average of 7.2 years and experienced some 45 impacts per derby and about 1900 impacts during their careers. They estimated speeds up to 50 kmph. When two cars rear-ended each other, impact increased further.

After the derby, fourteen drivers reported temporary musculoskeletal symptoms about the neck, shoulders, upper or lower back which lasted a few days in some drivers and one week in one driver.

Berry confirmed Melville's earlier observation on the lack of disability experienced by such drivers,[289] and noted, "The sports driver is not fearful or angered and is highly motivated to ignore minor symptoms, to continue with an active life, and to avoid the illness role, a difference that would account largely for the absence of chronic symptoms and disability."

Those who search for evidence in the whiplash mystery should pay close attention to the 31-year-apart observations of Melville and Berry.[289,290] Those who insist on a purely physical explanation for chronic whiplash symptoms must answer the question; why do car-crashing derby contestants with their repeated significant impacts have so little chronic disability?

Why have most researchers ignored Melville's vital contribution? [289,281] Why do they still ignore the 30 year reporting gap between North America and the UK?

A mystery indeed.

21

MORE EVIDENCE

Defining neck sprains or whiplash continued to lack consistency. In 1993, two Australians, J.R. Taylor and L.T. Twomey reported marked pathological changes in the cervical spines and intervertebral discs of 16 individuals who had died from severe trauma. Their study published in Spine[291] revealed the curious title, "Acute injuries to cervical joints. An autopsy study of neck sprain."

It is not possible to obtain autopsy results on persons with a neck sprain as such people do not die. The title made no sense. Taylor's patients died from horrendous head, chest or abdominal injuries or a combination of such injuries, not from sprained necks. Fourteen died in major automobile accidents, one was run over by a motor-cycle while lying in the road, while another died from hanging, - a strange addition to the paper.[291]

The pathological changes in these violently killed individuals cannot be considered relevant to living persons who experience common neck sprains following moderate impact motor vehicle collisions. Nevertheless, certain authorities quoted Taylor's work to support their claims that significant pathological changes in the cervical spine could occur among people who experienced common neck sprains following moderate automobile collisions.

For example, in the year 2000 physiatrist-teacher Dr. Robert Teasell from the University of Western Ontario, Canada[292] (the very same province from which Melville[289] had earlier described the lack of injury among car-crashing derby drivers!) teamed up with anatomist-researcher Dr. Nikolai Bogduk from the University of Newcastle, Australia, to quote Taylor's work in support of organic causes for whiplash symptoms, such as "tears of the annulus fibrosis" (of the cervical discs) and fractures or contusions of the zygapophyseal joints. (Joints in the cervical vertebrae) "These are the injuries found post-mortem in victims of fatal motor vehicle crashes."[292]

One year later Teasell, reviewing whiplash with psychiatrist Harold Merskey for the Trial Lawyers Association of British Columbia, again used Taylor and Twomey's study[291] to support organic causation in whiplash injury.[293] In a review, one normally presents a full spectrum of causation and treatment, but Teasell and Merskey, despite providing 103 references, avoided mentioning those suggesting psychosocial factors played a part in whiplash symptoms.

1. (2000) Henry Berry.[290] Canada.

Teasell was surely aware of Berry's work as it was published in the same issue of the <u>Archives of Neurology</u> as his own. [292] Berry, as noted earlier, found 14 of 20 demolition derby drivers to have experienced brief musculoskeletal symptoms following an average of 45 crashes at up to 50 kmph, but no symptoms lasting beyond one week. Berry, in his small sample, commented that the sports driver is highly motivated to ignore minor symptoms, continues with an active life and avoids the illness role.[290]

2. (1963) Melville.[289] Canada.

Earlier he observed 92 drivers in one derby with their heads in the large white helmets which are customary, "flailing through a great range of movement in response to the impacts involved". Inquiring from the pit steward at the track and later at the insurance company he learned of no reported injuries during this event and that serious injury in other events was extremely rare. The drivers enjoyed crashing their cars, the challenges and comradeship and avoided the treatment cycle.

3. (1986) Mills and Horne.[294] New Zealand.

Horne, an orthopedic surgeon, familiar with whiplash patients after practising in a large Eastern Canadian city, found such patients rare in Wellington, New Zealand where he practised later. Struck by the marked incidence difference in the two cities he compared, with the help of medical student Helen Mills, the frequency of whiplash in New Zealand with that of the state of Victoria, Australia, where there was a different insurance/legal system, patients seeking compensation through the common law. Horne and Mills found a reported incidence of whiplash injury ten times higher than that of New Zealand.[294,295]

4. (1992) Awerbach.[296] Australia.

He confirmed Horne's hypothesis that compensation reward affects reported whiplash incidence. After the Australian government changed the law in 1987, claimants had to report to police and pay the first $317. of any medical expense in whiplash injury claims. Claims in the state of Victoria immediately dropped from 6,364 in 1985/1986 to a mere 2004 the next year.

5. (1982) Balla.[297] Singapore.

Balla compared the frequency of whiplash in Australia with that of Singapore after directly interviewing neurosurgeons, neurologists and some orthopedic surgeons and psychiatrists. Chronic whiplash injury common in Australia was "virtually unheard of" in Singapore despite 90-100 car accidents occurring daily.

6. (1973) Farbman. 39 USA.

He studied 136 patients, referred from various sources with simple uncomplicated musculoligamentous neck sprain, searching for factors beside the accident which might influence recovery rate. He studied age, sex, race, occupation, marital status, habits, associated medical conditions, hospitalisation, x-ray findings, extent of car damage, emotional factors, extensiveness of past medical history, treatment and litigation.

Emotional factors prolonged symptoms the most. Extensive past medical history, overtreatment and litigation were other factors prolonging symptoms.

7. (1971) Macnab.[269] Canada.

Population sample. Examined 575 patients referred to him because of more severe difficulties following whiplash injury "whether physiogenically or psychogenically induced". Teasel included Macnab among his references but did not mention Macnab's noting of psychogenic factors among many patients.

8. (1964) Hodge.[37] USA.

Described four patients who suffered severe nervousness and psychological distress following whiplash injury, only one of whom did not report pre-existing psychosocial factors. Three reported being previously nervous for years. One gave a long past history of personal maladjustment and of multiple psychosomatic problems.

9. (1990) Malleson.[38] Canada.

Described 28 year-old history teacher Peter's experience. Apparently injured in a minor rear-end collision without vehicle damage six years earlier, he had not responded to "innumerable treatments" nor to a "host of medical experts." Prior to the accident he had experienced anxiety episodes while standing in front of his class, one of which caused acute chest pain requiring an emergency visit to hospital. He was a loner. Malleson noting that Peter had wasted six years of his life in invalidism, asked "can physicians and the law make compensation litigation less dangerous for others?"

10. (1993) Livingston.[279] Canada.

Searching the whiplash literature in 1992 he noted a long reporting gap between the United States and the UK.[272,277] Normally when a new syndrome is described in a major journal on one side of the Atlantic, it surfaces in a major journal on the other side within three years.

However, with whiplash such reporting was delayed a remarkable 30 years.[279] Livingston suggested that social factors including peer-copying among both patients and physicians could account for the reporting delay.

In another study he described the course of 101 consecutive unselected "whiplashed" patients in his general practice.[298] Patients were treated as in other sprains. Basic medication was offered and gentle exercising begun within one week of injury. No patients were referred for physiotherapy or chiropractic. 85 percent of patients recovered within six months and all within two years. The 15 patients whose symptoms lasted beyond six months had <u>problems pre-existing the accident;</u> physical such as severe osteoarthritis or spondylolisthesis, or psychosocial such as a history of many accidents, long standing neck or back pain in close family members, significant personal stress or overtreatment as in one patient who had apparently received more than 100 physiotherapy visits following a previous similar injury.

In later correspondence, Dr. Ian Macnab suggested that the comparatively good results described in the article were likely due to simplicity of treatment and lack of referral to other practitioners.

11. (1997) Ferrari and Russell.[299] Canada.

In an editorial for the <u>Journal of Rheumatology</u> stated, "we believe that the whiplash syndrome is an example of illness actually induced by society in general, and by physicians in particular. Common sense should tell us that a minor (indefinable) injury is not capable of generating the wide range of symptoms or the progressive deterioration over the first four months seen in this disorder."

They noted that rugby forwards occasionally encountered forces rendering them paraplegic but did not suffer whiplash-type injuries. They commented that overtreatment, continually restating their symptoms, keeping a daily diary at their lawyer's insistence, and multiple consultations with varied personnel all delayed whiplashed patients recovery.

12. (1998) Sullivan.[300] UK.

Sullivan, a British orthopedic surgeon, noted that the cost of litigation at the single patient level was usually twice as much as the award to the patient. He observed that in the adversarial system of litigation "it behoves each side to employ experts to write medical reports." This system took much time and it was not unusual for a simple whiplash injury case to be settled five years after the accident. Inevitably, both sides insisted on yearly updated medical reports; twenty-five percent of orthopedic surgeon's income came from such reports mostly following rear-end collisions. "Neither the medical nor legal professions wished to give up such remunerative acts."

The same pattern naturally occurs in North America among numerous experts in various disciplines producing a "starburst" of variable diagnoses,[290] and cases like Dr. Malleson's Peter in Chapter seven.[38] Speaking to the delighted trial lawyers Teasell and Merskey also attacked studies such as the Quebec Study[301], the Lithuanian Study[302] and the Saskatchewan Study[303] which suggested psychosocial and legal factors slowed recovery.

Many practitioners and lawyers prefer Teasell's organic explanation of pain. They have been trained to do so. Freeman,[304] a chiropractor at the University of Oregon, declared that a series of articles suggesting psychosocial reasons for chronic whiplash symptoms were "anecdotal evidence," or had "methodologic flaws." No doubt he would offer a similar opinion on our dozen reported research studies. However, the continued reporting of such studies should encourage practitioners to rethink the causes of chronic whiplash symptoms. Neurologist Berry stressed that,

"The clinician should be equally at ease with functional (behavioural) as well as physical diagnoses, and they must be given an equal-entity status. It may be inevitable, therefore, that some practitioners will never make a functional diagnosis."[290]

Interestingly, some fifty years earlier, poet-physician William Carlos Williams clearly noted the two types of diagnosis, - the physical and the psychosocial, among his patients in Rutherford, New Jersey.[34,144]

Recently, more evidence from Europe supports the earlier reports of Farbman, Berry, Melville, Horne and others. In 1999, Obelieniene, Schrader and colleagues followed up Schrader's earlier <u>Lancet</u> study[302]

with a prospective controlled inception cohort study of 210 consecutive persons experiencing rear-end collisions in Kaunas, Lithuania.[305] Forty-seven percent reported initial symptoms but one year later noted no more symptoms than a matched control sample of uninjured persons. Obelieniene and Schrader concluded that "where there was no preconceived notion of chronic pain following rear-end collisions, no fears of long-term disability and usually no involvement by therapists, insurance companies or lawyers, symptoms from whiplash injury' were brief and self-limiting." Partheni et al.[306] described a prospective study on 130 consecutive Greek patients having whiplash-associated disorder uncomplicated by fracture or neurological change, who received minimal or no therapy. Ninety-one percent were symptomless four weeks after their accident. Seemingly, this sample of Greeks like Melville's and Berry's[289,290] derby-drivers, considered their neck symptoms a minor matter.

Partheni declared "perhaps by not receiving (and then failing to respond to) multiple therapies, no anxiety is created. Patients do not change their activities to any extent, or stop work, and will not develop poor posture or poor physical fitness. Whiplash victims in Greece do not hear frightful diagnoses that mean to them chronic disability. In other countries, however, the media and medical community attention to whiplash enforces the notion that it causes chronic pain."[306]

Three years later in June to August 2002 the British Columbia Medical Journal published a series of articles on the whiplash syndrome.

Only one author, rheumatologist Dr. Robert Ferrari,[307] paid serious attention to Partheni's and Obelieniene's work. Physical causation for the whiplash syndrome was preferred. For example, J R Taylor[308] whose research was described at the start of this chapter, repeated his observations published in Spine[291] nine years earlier on the pathological changes in the cervical spine of dead victims of horrendous impact fatal car accidents. He still claimed that non-fatal moderate impact rear-end collisions could cause similar pathological changes.

Considering that Taylor's work was founded upon victims of fatal car accidents and not relevant to the mass of patients constantly visiting health practitioners and lawyers following moderate or minor collisions,[307,309,310], one wonders why his article was chosen for this whiplash series.

However, many physicians and others continue to prefer organic explanations of pain despite poor results in treating whiplash injury' as a purely physical matter. No wonder British Columbia has the highest incidence of whiplash in the world. [311,312]

We still do not know the pathological condition of the cervical spines in individual injured patients, but should we not learn from Lithuania and Greece where patients recover much quicker with fewer health practitioners, next to no lawyers, little insurance, minimal investigation and treatment and early return to their normal activities?

It is hard for patients who naturally attribute continuing symptoms to their accident. The lucky ones are listened to, carefully examined, receive reasonable explanation, avoid overtreatment and soon return to their usual activities.

In Western society practitioners, special clinics, lawyers and patients all appear to benefit financially from slowed recovery. Some practitioners have forgotten the basic Hippocratic principle,... "at least do no harm."[313]

Students can find more useful information in the earlier works of Ferrari, Malleson and Livingston.[282,283,311]

In the West the rising cost of health care causes increasing concern. Why do we ignore the increasing cost of treating whiplash? Perhaps because so many benefit from it. That, a narrow education and questionable research appear to be the main reasons for the whiplash mystery continuance.

Experts vary in their expertise. A specialty in orthopedics, rheumatology or psychiatry does not guarantee balanced expertness in whiplash type cases. Most orthopedic surgeons prefer operating to eliciting complex pain stories from whiplashed patients. They are trained for the former. Surely, it is more satisfying to replace an osteoarthritic hip and give a patient years of pain-free walking.

Rheumatologist Dr. Nortin Hadler after thorough education in the subtleties of rheumatology found he did not know how to advise a patient with backache.[314] His colleagues suggested he was "too productive a biochemist to trouble himself with such minor issues." Nevertheless, he determined to study musculoskeletal illness related to work incapacity.[314]

Modern medicine's continual division into subspecialties has encouraged individual doctors to have increased knowledge in some areas of their specialty, but less knowledge in others.

Many years ago I was privileged to hear neurosurgeon Dr. Peter Moyes give evidence on a neck injury case at the New Westminster Court house in British Columbia. I had just given my evidence and decided to stay to hear him. Dr. Moyes had the highest reputation as a neurosurgeon in British Columbia. There was no jury in this case and as Dr. Moyes continued his evidence the judge, obviously impressed by its quality, seized the opportunity to learn more and questioned him widely. In many instances Moyes replied, "We really don't know the answer to that, my Lord."

Would that all medical experts were that knowledgeable, honest and unbiased.

As I sat in the courtroom I thought how fortunate I was to hear Moyes' evidence and what a pity it was that a group of medical students was not present.

22

Always the Tale

We seem to have travelled in a circle. Two early cases encompassed four thousand years and represented the common spectrum of illness, from the purely physical disorder of the person whose sprained neck was described by the Egyptian surgeon in the introduction,[1] to Harriet's breathing problem in chapter one where the not-so-obvious cause was finally found to be psychosocial.

The Egyptian surgeon obtained the essential story from his patient - where the pain was and how it was aggravated; advised logical treatment, temporary support, medication and early movement restoration. Four thousand years later in Western society whiplashed patients often receive worse management amongst questionable research and continued debate.[315] For example, much-quoted Swiss psychiatrist Radanov and colleagues squeezed some 15 English language studies from the same patient sample they obtained by advertising - a serious selection bias. Kwan, Ferrari and Schrader noted numerous errors in their research.[315,316] Volume replaced accuracy.

However, researchers still quote Radanov as an authority. Why?

In Harriet's case five essentials were necessary for evaluation.

1. A home visit.

2. Her tale fully told, (chiefly by her husband.)

3. Her husband Bob, present in his familiar environment to offer his crucial diagnostic clue.

4. The practitioner needed to listen and to accept Bob's diagnosis.

5. Harriet needed to accept a psychosocial diagnosis as plausible.

The early chapters reveal that illness or injury may follow from physical factors, psychosocial factors or from a mix of both. In Harriet's case would a major tertiary-care medical centre have proven more effective than this basic home visit?

Katherine Hunter in her intriguing 1991 study, Doctors' Stories,[317] discussed the place of narrative (or the tale) in contemporary academic medicine. A Professor of Literature, she was invited to teach humanities to medical students and was given the opportunity to observe patients, students and staff in three Eastern United States teaching hospitals.

There she found narrative "nearly ignored." Pure biological and physical facts were emphasised in assessing patients, in writing up charts and in teaching ward rounds. Anecdotes were frowned upon. They were considered as "traps for their unwary auditors" who might mistake them for "real" knowledge.[317] As young physicians passed through their levels of residency such training habits were continuously reinforced. In streamlining the account of disease... "all narrative in medicine has been devalued...." (p.103)[317]

Scientific education is the principal purpose of the organised medical curriculum, and only science and scientifically-based clinical knowledge are consciously taught.[317]

Such devaluation of narrative would surely influence future specialists' later practice and actually discourage thorough listening. Interestingly, the great Swiss psychiatrist Carl Jung had deplored contemporary devaluation of the psyche and resistance to psychological enlightenment 40 years previously.[318]

Hunter did part of her investigation at the University of Rochester school of medicine and dentistry where Dr. George Engel, an internist with psychoanalytic training, was a staff member and where psychosocial issues were given some consideration. In 1980 Engel noted that "the dominant model in medicine today is called the biomedical model."[319] Engel suggested replacing that model with a new biopsychosocial model,' incorporating psychosocial factors to "fully encompass the human domain." He used a 'Medical' patient suffering from a heart attack to illustrate the importance of considering psychosocial issues in patient management.[319]

Later he described the weakness of the interrogative style of history-taking compared with simply encouraging patients to tell their story in their own way.[320] As we saw previously in our account, Michael Balint had used a similar approach earlier on the other side of the Atlantic.[32,33] In an editorial comment on Engel's article, Thomas Wise, editor of Psychosomatics, observed how in an era of managed care, shortened patient encounters, large group practices limiting a consistent primary care physician, and a reliance upon self-report inventories, it was easy to lose the essence of the doctor-patient relationship.[321]

Indeed, when taking a patient's history, an average of merely 18 seconds elapsed before one sample of doctors interrupted the patient's account.[322]

Howard Brody from Michigan illustrated the power of the anecdote by recounting a 12-year-old boy's experience.[323] The boy, angrily clinging to the belief that his father, a Vietnam veteran was still alive, had exhibited multiple behavioural problems at home and at school. During a "retreat" arranged for suffering families a researcher accompanied the boy for a walk in the woods. The boy "was his usual sullen and withdrawn self. Then they came upon a large dead tree, at the base of which a sapling grew. The boy stopped and stared at the tree for awhile, and the investigator was considerably surprised when the boy exclaimed, 'that tree makes me think of my father. You know, I realise now that my father is dead. I think he's that big tree and I'm the sapling. As it dies, the big tree loses its leaves, and lets the sunlight through so that the sapling can grow.'"

In one magical moment the untutored boy created a healing parable, accepted his father's death and his own continuing life and growth. No structured "history" was taken. (My underlining) True, the tale may be "a trap for the unwary,"[317] may be a lie (well-demonstrated in Dr. Williams's story, "The Use of Force")[134] or be affected by memory loss or exaggeration. Nevertheless even in its frailty the tale may prove revealing. Sir Richard Bayliss, while instructing medical students at a London teaching hospital on how to receive a history, described how the words tumble out.[324]

"In the clinical context the doctor has not only to hear and see the verbal and visual presentations but must record the essence of them. To the tidy-minded professional the temptation to interrupt the patient in order to clarify ambiguities or to obtain more details must be steadfastly resisted until the patient has finished. Histories must be received, not taken."

While interviewing 45-year-old Mrs. Trumper with four medical students, Bayliss described the events in a London hospital outpatient department.

"She smiled and her opening words were, 'I'm happily married but I have the most terrible headaches.' I stopped her because I wanted to see how many of the four students sitting with me had heard what she had said. I handed each of them a slip of paper and asked them to write down the patient's exact words.... Three recorded that Mrs Trumper had severe headaches, 'only one that she was happily married and had severe headaches.' None, apparently had noticed the smile on her face."

Bayliss asked the students why she said she was happily married before mentioning her headaches. It turned out (as we might suspect) that she was most unhappily married, a major factor in her headaches. He stressed that a careful history was the most important factor in discovering the diagnosis.

Hunter[325] noted that the patient-centered interview resists the enchantment of technology and goes a long way toward remedying the neglect of the sick person that has marred late twentieth-century medical care.

Today we are still dazzled by technology which has achieved so much in our modern world. It is easy to neglect listening and to neglect history. Yet past observers of human nature often achieved better balance between mind and body. Chekhov listened to his patients

tirelessly,[77] (chapter 11) and from his experience produced tales such
as Misery[73] and A Doctor's Visit[117] which reveal the diagnostic and
healing power of narrative. Williams (chapter 12) well understood
the psychosocial factors in illness.[130,131,134] He lost himself in the very
properties of his patients' minds.[144]

Historian Edward Shorter showed how patients' psychosomatic
symptoms developed during the past three centuries.[326] Certain
symptom patterns became popular in the 1700s, motor symptoms such
as fits, weakness and apparent paralyses, and sensory such as fatigue
and pain. For example:

"Bridget Byng, healthy enough to outlive her husband John - the
fifth Lord Torrington - by ten years was continuously ill throughout
the 1780s and early 1790s." Her husband commented in his diary on
his wife and her whole set: "All my ladies were so fatigued by the toil
of the day, that they hurried home to bed: a most precious, nervous set,
encouraging each other in sickness and fancies; never drinking one
glass of wine but by the advice of the doctor. The maids, in imitation
of their mistresses, fall sick likewise, and complain bitterly of their bad
health!!"[326]

Symptom patterns can be found earlier still in the beautiful words
of William Shakespeare. For example, in his play The First Part of
Henry IV published in 1598 Shakespeare describes the action between
Lady Percy and her husband Henry (Harry) Hotspur recently wounded
leading his soldiers in battle. Hotspur is reading a letter which warns
him against a plot he is considering. He is stressed and anxious. His
wife enters the room and complains bitterly about his behaviour. (Act
2, scene 3, line 30)[327]

Lady Percy. "O my good Lord, why are you thus alone?
For what offence have I this fortnight been
A banished woman from my Harry's bed?
Tell me, sweet Lord, what is't that takes from thee
Thy stomach, pleasure, and thy golden sleep?
Why dost thou bend thine eyes upon the earth
And start so often when thou sit'st alone?
Why hast thou lost the fresh blood in thy cheeks,
And given my treasures and my rights of thee

To thick-eyed musing and curst melancholy?
In thy faint slumbers I by thee have watched,
And heard thee murmur tales of iron wars...
  ...of soldiers slain,
And all the currents of a heady fight.
Thy spirit within thee hath been so at war,
And thus hath so bestirred thee in thy sleep,
That beads of sweat have stood upon thy brow..."
and so on.

Shakespeare captures the essence of anxiety-depression, aloneness, downcast eyes, jumpiness, avoiding intimacy with his wife, disordered stomach, diminished enjoyment, sleeplessness, talking of war in his sleep, his own spirit at war within him, beads of sweat upon his brow, "curst melancholy." She fears he does not love her.

Shakespeare, careful student of human nature, was well aware of the symptoms and that some of his audience would recognise the effects of a troubled mind upon the body. Incidentally, he presents a fuller description of anxiety-depression than Dr. Chekhov did in Ivanov 300 years later.[84] (chapter 11).

Shakespeare can still open minds. Indeed, we may find more truth in Shakespeare's narrative fiction than in many 'facts' of medical research.[328] Today, some doctors in our uncertain society would diagnose "chronic fatigue syndrome" or "fibromyalgia,"[329] contemporary names for ancient symptom patterns. Patients continue to copy symptoms and seek out special clinics where their disease may, in effect, be encouraged. The diseases enter the culture in which the patient lives, becoming fixed by copying, by the media, especially television, and by experts, few of whom realise they are repeating history.

Some critics argue that listening to patients takes too much time.[330] However, in many instances it saves both time and resources as can be seen by reviewing the four patients in chapter seven, Maria, Tanya, Mary and Gloria and the patients in Balint's book.[32]

As my teacher and friend, the late Dr. John Mennell used to say at every lecture I ever heard him give. "Listen to the patient. Listen to the patient. The patient is <u>trying to tell you</u> the diagnosis."

Not only is careful listening the first step to accurate diagnosis, it may prove to be the first step on the path toward healing.

Actually, we need more than a clinical diagnosis. In 1988, Hadler[331] described the focus upon disease rather than the patient in contemporary teaching hospitals, confirming observations by Balint, [33] Engel,[319] Hunter,[317] and Williams's two levels of diagnosis.[144,145]

"There is no time and little pretence to listen to these patients, and even less to know them. It will probably take decades to realise the tragedy of all this and then to become accustomed to offer an assessment of the patient rather than a 'diagnosis.'"[331]

Most medical care occurs outside teaching hospitals.[332] Who will describe it? Who will teach it? In chapter one we saw how the patient's husband diagnosed her personal experience of illness. The doctor simply acknowledged Bob's vital contribution. Our immediate need is for patients, primary care physicians, nurses and subspecialists to communicate better with one another and to appreciate each others' contributions and limits.

Traditional family doctors[333-335] especially have the opportunity to build patients' trust over the years, strengthening health care through their continuing actions and through listening. We need more outspoken generalists. In the sixties people wanted generalists, but were encouraged toward fragmented costly multi-specialists who achieved greater status. Today, in Canada's deteriorating "health system" many cannot find a personal family doctor. A significant loss. Family doctors can treat more than 80 percent of health problems and can provide continuing care. Patients' tales must be recorded, published, read, and understood. History slips away every second.

Treasure the tale.

TABLE 1

Canadian G.P. Researchers   1954-1969

Year	Author	Age	Town	popn (000s)	Size of Practice	Medical School
'54	Walsh, AC	36	Vancouver, BC	366	2	Alberta, 1943
'56	Coleman J	47	Duncan, BC	25	3	Toronto, 1935
'57	Anderson,W	47	Kelowna, BC	30	7	McGill, 1935
'59	Malkin,S	43	Winnipeg, Man	200	Solo	Manitoba, 1940
'60	Cauchon R	52	Donnaconna, Que	5	Solo	Laval, 1932
'62	Brook, M	51	Saskatoon, Sask	95	2	Manitoba, 1935
'62	Fogel,S	42	Saskatoon, Sask	95	Solo	Edinburgh, 1952
'63	McWilliam R	40	Stratford, Ont	23	3	Edinburgh, 1945
'63	Brown,D	30	Amhurst, NS	10	Solo	Dalhousie, 1959
'64	Wolfe,S	41	Saskatoon, Sask.	115	~10	Toronto, 1950
'64	McAnulty J	35	Oyama & Winfield, BC	2	Solo	Edinburgh, 1957
'65	Lane,R	37	Chilliwack, BC	25	3	Toronto, 1953
'65	Glen, N	42	Amherst, NS	10	2	Bristol, 1947
'67	Malyska,W	49	Deloraine, Man	1	2	Manitoba, 1939
'67	Paul, M	36	Toronto, Ont	664	Solo	Toronto, 1957
'67	Bain, S	38	Toronto, Ont	664	~10	Toronto, 1953
'68	Scott,F	36	Loon Lake, Sask	0.8	Solo	Durham, 1956
'68	Livingston M	40	Richmond, BC	58	Solo	Alberta, 1953
'69	McFarlane A	37	Hamilton, Ont	290	5	Queen's, 1957
'69	Westbury R	33	Calgary, Alta	400	5	Cambridge, 1963
'69	Lawee, D	40	Toronto, Ont	664	6	Paris, 1953

SELECTED BIBLIOGRAPHY

1. BREASTED JH. The Edwin Smith Surgical Papyrus, Vol. 1. Hieroglyphic Transliteration, Translation and Commentary. Chicago, University of Chicago Press, 1930, p.452-454.

2. MEALY K, BRENNAN H, & FENELON GCC. "Early mobilisation of acute whiplash injuries." Br Med J 1986; 292:656-657.

3. SPITZER WO, SKOVRON L, SALMI LR et al. Scientific Monograph of the Quebec Task Force on Whiplash-Associated Disorders. Spine 1995;20: Supp S 36.

4. HIPPOCRATES. Epidemics 111. In Hippocrates (Jones WHS, transl.) London, William Heinemann, 1923, Vol 1. p.231-233.

5. HIPPOCRATES. Epidemics 1. In The Genuine Works of Hippocrates, (Adams F. transl.) London, The Sydenham Society, 1849, Vol. 1. p.352-353.

6. MILLER GL. "Literacy and the Hippocratic Art: Reading, writing and epistemology in ancient Greek medicine." J Hist Med 1990; 45:11-40.

7. SHORTER E. From Paralysis to Fatigue, a History of Psychosomatic Illness in the Modern Era. New York, The Free Press, 1992.

8. WILLIAMS WC. The Autobiography of William Carlos Williams. New York, New Directions, 1967, p. 356.

9. SACKS O. The Man Who Mistook His Wife for a Hat. London, Duckworth & Co, 1985, p. 7-21.

10. LOCKWOOD A.L. in GROVES A. "All in the Day's work." Toronto, Macmillan Company of Canada, 1933, Foreword ix-xiv.

11. TALBOTT J.H. A Biographical History of Medicine, New York, Grune and Stratton, 1970, p. 560.

12. HANCOCK H. "Disease of the Appendix Calci cured by operation." Address to the Medical Society of London, Lancet, 1848; 11:380.

13. SINGER C and UNDERWOOD E.A. A Short History of Medicine. Oxford, Clarendon Press, 1962, p. 365.

14. GROVES A. All in the Day's Work. Toronto, Macmillan Company of Canada, 1934, p. 20.

15. GROVES A. Ibid. p. 8.

16. GROVES A. Ibid. p. 15

17. POWER, D. "Treves' first appendix operation." Brit J Surg 1935; 23:1.

18. HIPPOCRATES. Articulations. In the Genuine Works of Hippocrates. Vol. 1. (Adams F. Transl.) London, The Sydenham Society, 1849; p.612.

19. HIPPOCRATES. Articulations. ibid, p.606.

20. CYRIAX J. Textbook of Orthopaedic Medicine. Vol. 1. London, Bailliére Tindall, 8th Ed. 1982, p.148.

21. EBERLE J. A Treatise on the Practice of Medicine. Vol. 1. 2nd Ed. Philadelphia, John Grigg, 1831, p. 382.

22. PAGET J. "Cases that Bone-setters Cure." Brit Med J 1867;1:1-4.

23. LIVINGSTON M. "Spinal Manipulation causing injury: a three year study." Clin Orthop 1971;81:82-86.

24. CURTIS P and BOVE G. "Family physicians, chiropractors and back pain." J Fam Pract 1992;35:551-555.

25. DAVIS EH, BEASLEY JW, KELLY MJ, ABEND DS and CHERKIN, D. "Chiropractic." [Letters] J Fam Pract 1993; 36: 378-379.

26. LIVINGSTON M. "Chiropractic by FP's." [Letter] J Fam Pract 1993; 37:117.

27. LEE P, CARLINI WG, McCORMICK GF and ALBERS GW. "Neurologic complications following chiropractic manipulation: a survey of California neurologists." Neurology 1995; 45:1213-1215.

28. FRISONI GB and NAZOLA GP. "Vertebrobasilar ischemia after neck motion." Stroke 1991; 22:1452-1460.

29. MARTIN GM. "Sprain, strain and whiplash injury." Phys Ther 1959; 39:803-813.

30. BARNSLEY L, LORD S, BOGDUK N. "Whiplash injury." Pain 1994;58:283-307.

31. SARNO JE. "Etiology of neck and back pain: an autonomic myoneuralgia?" J Nerv Ment Dis 1981; 169: 55-59.

32. BALINT M. The Doctor, His Patient And The Illness. 2nd Ed. Edinburgh, Churchill Livingstone, 1986, p. 119.

33. BALINT M. Ibid. P. 121.

34. WILLIAMS WC. The Autobiography of William Carlos Williams. New York, New Directions Publishing Corporation, P. 358, 356, 361, 362.

35. BALINT M. Ibid. p.15-20.

36. ELLARD J. "Psychological reactions to compensatable injury." Med J Aust 1970; 2:349-355.

37. HODGE JR. "The Whiplash injury: A discussion of this phenomenon as a psychosomatic illness." Ohio Med J 1964;60: 762-766.

38. MALLESON A. "Whiplash: folly and fakery." Humane Med 1990;6:193-196.

39. FARBMAN AA. "Neck sprain. Associated factors." JAMA 1973; 223:1010-1015.

40. ACKERNECHT EH. Rudolph Virchow:Doctor, Statesman, Anthropologist. Madison, University of Wisconsin Press, 1953.

41. ACKERNECHT EH. Ibid. p. 132-135.

42. REESE DM. "Fundamentals-Rudolph Virchow and modern medicine." West J Med 1998; 169:105-8.

43. BALINT M. Ibid. p. 129.

44. BALINT M. Ibid. p. 21-36.

45. BALINT M. Ibid. p. 41.

46. BALINT M. Ibid. p. 42.

47. BALINT M. Ibid. p.43.

48. BALINT M. Ibid. p.25,29.

49. HADLER N. Occupational Musculoskeletal Disorders, New York, Raven Press, 1993, p. 18-20.

50. HADLER N. Ibid. p. 28.

51. BALINT M. Ibid. p. 81-83.

52. FLEETCROFT R. "The General Physician-extinction or evolution." J Roy Soc Med (Editorial) 1998:91; 613.

53. SACKS O. Ibid, Preface X.

54. LIVINGSTON M. "Whiplash injury: why are we achieving so little?"

J Roy Soc Med 2000;93:526-529.

55. MACAULAY TB. History of England. Boston, Houghton 1899.

56. BARON J. The Life of Edward Jenner. M.D. London, 1827.

57. FISK DM. Dr. Jenner of Berkeley. London, Heinemann. 1959.

58. GIBSON WC. Creative Minds in Medicine. Springfield, Illinois, Charles E. Thomas, 1963, P. 150-153.

59. JENNER E. An Inquiry into the Causes and Effects of the Variolae Vaccinae. London, S Low, 1798.

60. HUNTINGTON G. "On chorea." Med Surg Rep 1872: 26; 317.

61. OSLER W. The Principles and Practice of Medicine. New York, D Appleton & Co, 1893.

62. SIMON RP, AMINOFF MJ, GREENBERG DA. Clinical Neurology. Appleton & Lange, Stamford CT, 1999, p. 242-243.

63. HARDING AE. "Movement Disorders" in Brain's Diseases of the Nervous System 10th Ed.(Ed. John Walton) Oxford, Oxford University Press, 1993, p. 414.

64. VESSIER PR. "On the transmission of Huntington's chorea for 300 years: The Bures Family group." J Nerv Ment Dis 1932:76; 553.

65. SIMMONS EJ. Chekhov. A Biography. Boston, Little, Brown and Company, 1962, p.6.

66. TROYAT H. Chekhov. New York, Random House, Ballantine Books, 1988, p. 16.

67. SIMMONS EJ. Ibid. p. 32.

68. COOPE J. Doctor Chekhov: A Study in Literature and Medicine. Isle of Wight, Cross Publishing, 1997, p.18.

69. COOPE J. Ibid. p. 21.

70. TROYAT H. Ibid. p.43.

71. CHEKHOV A. "Letter to Nikolai Leykin," August 21, 1883, in Letters of Anton Chekhov. (Heim MH and Karlinsky S, Transl.) New York, Harper and Row, 1973, p. 41.

72. MILES P. and PITCHER H. Chekhov. The Early Stories 1883-88. London, John Murray, 1982, p. 37-40.

73. CHEKHOV A. Anton Chekhov's Short Stories. (Ed. Matlaw RE) New York, WW Norton & Company, 1979, p.12-16.

74. TROYAT H. Ibid. p.41.

75. TROYAT H. Ibid. p. 42.

76. COOPE J. Ibid. p. 21.

77. COOPE J. Ibid. p. 27.

78. TROYAT H. Ibid. p. 51.

79. TROYAT H. Ibid. p. 59.

80. TROYAT H. Ibid. p. 62.

81. KARLINSKY S. in Letters of Anton Chekhov, ibid. p. 53.

82. TROYAT H. Ibid. p. 71.

83. CHEKHOV A. "Letter to Dimitry Gigorovich," March 28, 1886, Letters of Anton Chekhov, ibid. p. 58-59.

84. CHEKHOV A. The Oxford Chekhov. vol 11. Platinov, Ivanov, The Seagull. Hingley R. trans and ed. Oxford University Press, Oxford, 1967, p. 172.

85. CHEKHOV A. "Letter to Suvorin," December 30, 1888, in Letters of Anton Chekhov, ibid. p. 75-83.

86. CHEKHOV A. The Oxford Chekhov. vol 11. ibid. p. 208.

87. CHEKHOV A. "Letter to Alexander Chekhov," November 20, 1887, in Letters of Anton Chekhov, ibid. p. 72-73.

88. HINGLEY R. Chekhov: a Biographical and Critical Study. London, George Allen and Unwin Ltd, 1966, p. 84-86.

89. CHEKHOV A. "Letter to Dimitry Grigorovich," January 12, 1888. in Letters of Anton Chekhov, ibid p. 91-94.

90. TROYAT H. Ibid. p. 19.

91. TROYAT H. Ibid. p. 93.

92. TROYAT H. Ibid. p. 98.

93. CHEKHOV A. "Letter to Alexei Suvorin," September 11, 1888, in Letters of Anton Chekhov, ibid. p. 107.

94. CHEKHOV A. "Letter to Alexei Suvorin," March 9, 1890, in Letters of Anton Chekhov, ibid. p. 158-161.

95. KARLINSKY S. In Letters of Anton Chekhov, ibid, p. 153.

96. SIMMONS EJ. Ibid. p. 222.

97. CHEKHOV A. Letter to MP Chekhov, 23-26 June, 1890. In a Journey to Sakhalin. (Brian Reeve. Transl.) Cambridge, England, Ian Faulkner Publishing, 1993, p. 385.

98. COOPE J. Ibid. p. 58.

99. CHEKHOV A. "Letter to Suvorin," June 27, 1890, in Letters of Anton Chekhov, Ibid, p. 169.

100. CHEKHOV A. A Journey to Sakhalin. (Brian Reeve, Transl.) Cambridge, England, Ian Faulkner Publishing, 1993, p. 132.

101. TROYAT H. Ibid. p. 127.

102. TROYAT H. Ibid. p. 128-129.

103. CHEKHOV A. A Journey To Sakhalin, Ibid. p. 92-100.

104. CHEKHOV A. A Journey to Sakhalin, Ibid. p. 97.

105. COOPE J. Ibid. p. 63.

106. COOPE J. Ibid. p. 96.

107. CHEKHOV A. A Journey to Sakhalin, Ibid, p. 24.

108. TROYAT H. Ibid. p. 159.

109. COOPE J. Ibid. 106.

110. COOPE J. Ibid. 118.

111. CHEKHOV, A. A Journey to Sakhalin, Ibid. p. 26.

112. KARLINSKY S. In Letters of Anton Chekhov, Ibid. p. 272.

113. HINGLEY R. "The Seagull" in The Oxford Chekhov, vol 11. Ibid. p. 256.

114. CHEKHOV A. The Undiscovered Chekhov: 38 New Stories. (Peter Constantine. Transl.) New York, Seven Stories Press, 1998.

115. CHEKHOV A. "Letter to Grigory Rossolimo," October 11, 1899. In Letters of Anton Chekhov, Ibid. p. 365.

116. CHEKHOV A. "Letter to Alexei Pleshcheyev," October 4, 1888. In Letters of Anton Chekhov, Ibid. p. 109.

117. CHEKHOV A. Anton Chekhov's Short Stories. Ibid. p. 202-211.

118. WILLIAMS WC. The Autobiography of William Carlos Williams. New York, New Directions Publishing Corp, 1951, p. 50-55.

119. MARIANI P. William Carlos Williams: A New World Naked. New York, McGraw-Hill Book Company, 1981, p. 29-30.

120. WILLIAMS WC. The Autobiography, Ibid. p. 47.

121. MIRIANI P. William Carlos Williams Ibid. p. 74-5.

122. WILLIAMS WC. The Selected Poems of William Carlos Williams. New York, New Directions Publishing Corporation, 1969, p.30.

123. WILLIAMS WC. The Autobiography. Ibid. p. 288-289.

124. ELIOT TS. The Waste Land. Collected Poems 1909-1912. London, Faber and Faber, 1963, p.61.

125. WILLIAMS WC. Selected Poems. Ibid. p. 67.

126. WILLIAMS WC. Selected Poems. Ibid. p. 91.

127. WILLIAMS WC. Selected Poems. Ibid. p. 26.

128. WILLIAMS WC. Selected Poems. Ibid. p. 94.

129. JARELL R. Introduction, in Selected Poems. Ibid. p. xvii.

130. WILLIAMS WC. The Autobiography. Ibid. p. 149.

131. WILLIAMS WC. The Autobiography. Ibid. p. 247.

132. WILLIAMS WC. The Autobiography. Ibid. p. 179.

133. WILLIAMS WC. The White Mule. New York, New Directions Publishing Corp. 1937.

134. WILLIAMS WC. The Doctor Stories. New York, New Directions Publishing Corp. 1932. p. 56-60.

135. WILLIAMS WC. The Doctor Stories. Ibid. p. 13-41.

136. COLES R. Introduction. In WILLIAMS WC. The Doctor Stories. Ibid. p. vii-xvi.

137. COLES R. "William Carlos Williams: A Writing Physician." JAMA 1981; 245:41-42.

138. WILLIAMS WC. The Autobiography. Ibid. p. 311.

139. MARIANI P, William Carlos Williams. Ibid. p. 365.

140 COLES R. Introduction. In WILLIAMS WC. The Doctor Stories. Ibid. p. xiv.

141. WILLIAMS WC. "Paterson" The Autobiography. Ibid. p. 390.

142. WILLIAMS WC. The Autobiography. Ibid. p. 286.

143. MARIANI P. William Carlos Williams. Ibid. p. 768.

144. WILLIAMS WC. The Autobiography. Ibid. p. 356-362.

145. COLES R. Introduction. In WILLIAMS WC. The Doctor Stories. Ibid. p. xv.

146. PICKLES WN. Epidemiology in Country Practice. Re-Issued. Torquay, Devon. The Devonshire Press Ltd. 1972, p. 1-4. 89-107.

147. PICKLES WN. "Bornholm Disease: Acount of a Yorkshire Outbreak."

Brit Med J 1933;3:817.

148. SYLVEST E. "La maladie de Bornholm," Bull off int Hyg publ 1932; 24:1431.

149. CRONE NL and CHAPMAN EM. "Epidemic Pleurodynia," New Engl J Med 1933; 209:1007.

150. HUNT JH. Introduction, Epidemiology in Country Practice, 1973, vii-xiii.

151. Harrison's Principles of Internal Medicine. Ed's. FAUCI AS, BRAUNWALD E, ISSELBACHER KJ, WILSON JD, MARTIN JB, KASPER DL, HAUSER SL, LONGO DL. 14th Ed, Vol. 1. 1998, p.1122.

152. GIBSON WC. Creative Minds in Medicine. Springfield, Ill., Charles C. Thomas,1963, p. 153-5.

153. CASTIGLIONI A. A History of Medicine. New York, Alfred Knopf, 1941. p. 808-9.

154. GIBSON WC. Ibid. p. 155-6.

155. CASTIGLIONI A. Ibid. p. 620-1.

156. WITHERING W. An Account of the Foxglove. (1785.) In Mann RD. William Withering and the foxglove. Lancaster, England, MTP press ltd, 1985, p. 127-172.

157. MAIR A. Sir James Mackenzie M.D. 1853-1925. General Practitioner. Edinburgh, Churchill Livingstone, 1973, p. 9.

158. MAIR A. Ibid. p. 36.

159. MAIR A. Ibid. p. 47.

160. WILSON RM. The Beloved Physician. Sir James Mackenzie. London, John Murray, 1926, p. 172.

161. MAIR A. Ibid. p. 110.

162. MAIR A. Ibid. p. 113.

163. MAIR A. Ibid. p. 118.

164. WILSON RM. The Beloved Physician. Ibid. p. 55.

165. MACKENZIE J. Diseases of the Heart. London. Hodder & Stoughton, 1908, p.142-159.

166. MACKENZIE J. Ibid. p. 158.

167. MACKENZIE J. "The cause of heart irregularity in influenza with a demonstration of the clinical polygraph." Brit Med J 1902;11:1411.

168. MACKENZIE J. The Study of the Pulse. Edinburgh, Young J Pentland, 1902.

169. MACKENZIE J. The Study of the Pulse. Ibid. p. x.

170. MAIR A. Ibid. p. 129.

171. MAIR A. Ibid. Appendix. p. 348.

172. GIBSON WC. Creative Minds in Medicine. Ibid. p. 160.

173. MOORHEAD R. "Sir James Mackenzie (1853-1925): views on general practice education and research." J Roy Soc Med 1999; 92:38-43.

174. MACKENZIE J. Diseases of the Heart. Ibid. p. 42-51.

175. WILSON RM. The Beloved Physician. Ibid. p. 220.

176. HOWIE JGR. "Addressing the credibility gap in general practice research: better theory; more feeling; less strategy." Brit J Gen Pract. 1996; 46:479-81.

177. MAIR A. Ibid. p. 150.

178. CHEKHOV A. "Letter to Maria Kiselyova," January 14, 1887, in Letters of Anton Chekhov. Ibid. p. 60-64.

179. BRASSET EA. A Doctor's Pilgrimage. Philadelphia, J.B. Lippincott Company, 1951, p. 27-31.

180. BRASSET EA. Ibid. p. 39-41.

181. BRASSET EA. Ibid. p. 52-55.

182. CHATENAY H. The Country Doctors. Red Deer, Alberta, Matrix Press, 1980, p. 61-66.

183. HUME M. Prologue. In HUME M. with THOMMASEN H. River of the Angry Moon. Vancouver, Greystone Books and Seattle, University of Washington Press, 1998. p. i-iii.

184. WOOLARD RF and OSTRY AS. Eds. Fatal Consumption. Rethinking Sustainable Development. Vancouver, UBC Press, 2000.

185. GUNN CC, ISLIP MC, MASTERS DL, ESKINE-MURRAY H, RIGG CA & STAPLETON T. Arch Dis Child. "Iron-Deficency Anaemia between 3 months and 2 years of age, a comparision of treatment with ferrous sulphate and ferrous fumerate." 1959; 35: 281-284.

186. GUNN CC, MILBRANDT WE. "Tenderness at motor points: a diagnostic and prognostic aid for low-back injury." J Bone Joint Surg 1976; 58A:815-825.

187. GUNN CC, MILBRANDT WE. "Tennis elbow and the cervical spine." Can Med Assoc J 1978;114:803-809.

188. AXELSSON J, THESSLEFF S. "A Study of supersensitivity in denervated mammalian skeletal muscles." J Physiol 1959;147:178-193.

189. GUNN CC, MILBRANDT WE. "Early and subtle signs in low-back sprain." Spine 1978;3:267-281.

190. GUNN CC, MILBRANDT WE, LITTLE AS, MASON KE. "Dry-needling of muscle motor points for chronic low back pain. A randomised clinical trial with long term follow-up." Spine 1980;5:179-291.

191. LEWIT K. "The needle effect in the relief of myofascial pain." Pain 1978;6:83-90.

192. CANNON WB, ROSENBLUETH A. The Supersensitivity of Denervated Structures. New York, The Macmillan Company, 1949, 1-22, 185.

193. GUNN CC. " 'Prespondylosis' and some pain syndromes following denervation supersensitivity." Spine 1980;5:185-192.

194. GUNN CC. The Gunn Approach to the Treatment of Chronic Pain. New York, Churchill Livingstone, 1989.

195. GUNN CC. Treatment of Chronic Pain. Ibid. p. 6.

196. LOESER JD, CHAPMAN CR, BUTLER S, SOLA AE. In GUNN, CC. Treatment of Chronic Pain 1989. Ibid. p. VII.

197 WALL PD. Foreword in GUNN CC. Treatment of Chronic Pain. Ibid. p IX.

198. LIVINGSTON PC. Fringe of the Clouds. Toronto, The Ryerson Press, 1962.

199. LIVINGSTON PC. Ibid. p. 149 - 177.

200. LIVINGSTON PC. Ibid. p. 194-210.

201. LIVINGSTON MCP. "Spinal manipulation in medical practice: A century of ignorance." Med J Aust 1968; 2:552-255.

202. GREEN D and JOYNT RJ. " Vascular accidents to the brain stem associated with neck manipulation." JAMA 1959; 170:522-524.

203. PRATT-THOMAS HR and BERGER DE. "Cerebellar and spinal injuries after chiropractic manipulation." JAMA 1947; 133:600-603.

204. TERRETT AGJ. 'Vascular accidents from cervical spine manipulation." J Aust Chiropractors' Assoc 1987; 17:15-24.

205. WENTE M "Horrible Chiropractic Hazards." Globe and Mail Toronto, Canada April 23, 2002.

206. LIVINGSTON MCP. "Spinal Manipulation: Follow-up study of 60 patients." Manual Med 1970; 3: 59-62.

207. LIVINGSTON MCP. "Research and the Canadian general practitioner." The Practitioner 1971; 206:675-680.

208. LIVINGSTON MCP. "The background of some Canadian general practitioner-observers." Can Med Ass J 1971; 106:797-799.

209. LIVINGSTON MCP. "Observations on family practice research."

Can Family Physician May 1973; 19:106-108.

210. LIVINGSTON MCP. "Researching Recent Researchers." Can Family Physician 1974; 20:84-89.

211. McWHINNEY IR. "Advances in General Practice." The Practitioner 1969;203:535.

212. WALSH AC. "The use of local anaesthetic with a tourniquet in surgery of the hand." Can Med Ass J 1954;70:539-541.

213. COLEMAN JV. "Adenocarcinoma of the common bile duct." Can Med Ass J 1956;75:576-579.

214. ANDERSON WF. "Blighted twin." Can Med Ass J 1953;216:218.

215. MALKIN S. "Oral versus parenteral penicillin." Can Med Ass J 1959;81:553-557.

216. CAUCHON R. "Coxsackie epidemic." Bull Coll Gen Pract Can 1960;7:23-25.

217. BROOK MH and BROOK J. "Emergency Resuscitation." Brit Med J 1962; 2:1564-1566.

218. FOGEL S and HOFFER A. "Perceptual changes induced by hypnotic suggestion for the posthypnotic state. J Clin Exp Psychopath 1962; 23:24-35.

219. McWILLIAM RS, MacDONALD A and LINDSAY I. "Thrombophlebitis following the use of Norethynodrel (Enovid)." Can Med Ass J 1963; 88:1032-1033.

220. BROWN DC. "Congenital biliary atresia in identical twins." NS Med Bull 1963; 42:181-185.

221. WOLFE S. "Saskatchewan's community clinics." Can Med Ass J 1964; 91;225-229.

222. McANULTY J. "Sleepy Lagoon." Can Med Ass J 1964; 91:1064-1071.

223. LANE RF. "A cervical cytology program in general practice." Can Med Ass J 1965; 92:1203-1206.

224. GLEN NG. "Towards more and better family doctors." NS Med Bull 1965; 44:85-94.

225. MALYSKA W and CHRISTENSEN J. "Autohypnosis and the prenatal class." Am J Clin Hyp 1967; 9:188-192.

226. PAUL MM. "Interval therapy with dimethyl sulfoxide." Ann NY Acad Sci 1967; 141:586-598.

227. BAIN ST and SPAULDING WB. "The importance of coding presenting symptoms." Can Med Ass J 1967;97:953-959.

228. SCOTT F and MILLER MJ. "Trials with Metronidizole in amoebic dysentery." JAMA 1970; 211:118-120.

229. McFARLANE AH and O'CONNELL BP. "Morbidity in family practice." Can Med Ass J 1969; 101:259-263.

230. WESTBURY RC and TARRANT M. "Classification of disease in general practice; A comparative study." Can Med Ass J 1969;101:82-87.

231. LAWEE D. "Primary tuberculosis inguinal lymphadenitis." Can Med Ass J 1969;100:34-36.

232. FLEXNER A. "Medical education in the United States and Canada." Bulletin No. 4, Carnegie Foundation for the advancement of teaching. New York, 1910, 7-15.

233. BARDEEN CR. "Modern Praeceptors." JAMA 1928; 90:1177-1181.

234. SIVERTSON SE, STONE HL. "Is the Praeceptorship an anachronism?" JAMA 1972; 221:590-592.

235. PHILLIPS TJ, SWANSON AG. "Teaching Family Medicine in Rural Clinical Clerkships." A WAMI progress report. JAMA 1974; 228:1408-1410.

236. MILLIS JS. Report of the Citizens Commission on Graduate Medical Education. Sponsored by the American Medical Association. 1966, Chicago, Illinois.

237. Meeting the Challenge of Family Practice. Report of the Ad Hoc Committee on Education for Family Practice of the Council on Medical Education. American Medical Association 1966. Chicago, Illinois.

238. Report by the National Commission on Community Health Services. Health is a Community Affair. 1966.

239. LIVINGSTON MCP, MD., BASS S, MSc., EMERY AW, MD., THOMSON TA, BSc., YOUNGASH RN, BSc., and ZACK PS, BSc. "Six medical students in a community hospital." Can Med Ass J 1973; 109:1013-1016.

240. LIVINGSTON MCP, MD., THOMSON TA, BSc., VAUGHAN GA, BSc., BASS S, BSc., LEE HPK, BSc., MALPASS PB, BSc., WONG WTY, BSc., YOUNGASH RN BSc., and ZACK PS, BSc. "Medical students in community physicians offices." Can Med Ass J 1974;111:969-971.

241. PETERSON OL, ANDREWS LP, SPAIN RS, et al. "An analytical study of North Carolina general practice 1953-1954."J Med Educ 1956;31:1-165.

242. CLUTE KF. The General Practitioner. A Study of Medical Education and Practice in Ontario and Nova Scotia. Toronto, U of Toronto Press, 1963.

243. MYCKATYN MM, MILES JE. "A profile of today's medical student." Can Med Ass J 1973; 109;1118-1122.

244. LIVINGSTON MCP, EMERY AW, MacLACHLAN RG. "Student acceptance of two family practice teaching programs." Can Fam Phys 1975; 21:114-116.

245 SEDAL L. "Medical Education." Med J Aust 1972;11:1081-1085.

246. BALINT. Ibid. p. 91.

247. LLOYD G. "Montreal and Manchester: Their approaches to Family Practice." Can Fam Phys 1974; 20:71-73.

248. STEPHENS GG. The Intellectual Basis of Family Practice. Winter Publishing Company Inc. Tucson, Arizona, 1982.

249. Report of the Citizens Commission on Graduate Medical Education. Ibid. p.42.

250. Report of the Citizens Commission. Ibid. p. 39.

251. LEONE-PERKINS M, SCHNUTH RL, LIPSKY MS. "Students' evaluation of teaching and learning experiences at Community - and Residency -based practices." Fam Med 1999; 31:572-577.

252. General Medical Council. Tomorrow's Doctors: Recommendations on Under-graduate Medical Education. London. G M C, 1993.

253. COLEMAN K, MURRAY E. "Patients´ views and feelings on the community-based teaching of undergraduate medical students: a qualitative study." Family Practice 2002; 19:813-188.

254. MURRAY E, MODELL M. "Community-based teaching:the challenges." Brit J Gen Pract 1999;49:395-398.

255. FERENCHICK GS, CHAMBERLAIN J, ALGUIRE P. "Community-based teaching: Defining the added value for students and preceptors." Am J Med 2002; 112:512-517.

256. WHITE KL, WILLIAMS TF, GREENBERG BG. "The Ecology of Medical Care." N Eng J Med 1961; 265:885-892.

257. LIVINGSTON MC. "Some facets of alternative medicine-today and yesterday." West J Med 1985: 143:269-270.

258. EISENBERG DM KESSLER RC FOSTER C NORLOCK FE et al. "Unconventional medicine in the United States – Prevalence, costs and patterns of use." N Eng J Med 1993; 328:246-252

259. BARRETT S. "'Alternative' Medicine" More Hype than Hope." In Alternative Medicine and Ethics. Eds. JH HUMBER and ROBET F ALMEDER. HUMANA PRESS Inc. TOWATA, NJ, 1988, p. 1-42.

260. PATEL V. "Understanding the Integration of Alternative Modalities into an Emerging Healthcare Model in the United States."

In Alternative Medicine and Ethics. Eds. JH HUMBER and ROBERT F ALMEDER. HUMANA PRESS Inc. TOWATA, NJ, 1988, p. 43-95.

261. KAPTCHUK TJ, EISENBERG DM. "Varieties of healing 2: A taxonomy of unconventional healing practices." Ann Int Med 2001; 135:196-204.

262. ERNST E. "Harmless Herbs? A review of the recent literature." Am J Med 1998; 104:170-78

263. BISHOP M. "Should doctors be the judges of medical orthodoxy? The Barker Case." J Roy Soc Med 2002; 95:41-45.

264. BALINT M. Ibid. p. 1-8, 116, 172-3.

265. THOMAS L. The medusa and the snail: more notes of a biology watcher. New York: Viking Press, 1979, p. 47.

266. GREENHALGH T AND HURWITZ B. "Why study narrative?" In Narrative Based Medicine. (Eds. Trisha Greenhalgh and Brian Hurwitz) London, BMJ Books, 1998, p. 9,10.

267. WOODS D. "A conversation with Norman Cousins." (Interview). Can Med Assoc J 1983; 128:110-1113.

268. SIGERIST HE. Primitive and Archaic Medicine. Vol 1, in A History of Medicine. Oxford University Press, 1951, p. 267.

269. MACNAB I. "The 'Whiplash Syndrome.'" Orthop Clin North Am 1971;2:389-403.

270. CROWE HE. "Injuries to the cervical spine." Paper presented at the meeting of the Western Orthopedic Association, San Francisco, 1928.

271. DAVIS AG. "Injuries of the cervical spine." JAMA 1945; 127:149-156.

272. GAY JR and ABBOTT KH. "Common whiplash injuries of the neck." JAMA 1953; 152:1698-1704.

273. PENNIE B and AGAMBAR L. "Patterns of injury and recovery in whiplash." Injury 1991;22:57-60.

274. MCCONNELL WE, VANPOPPEL J, KRAUSE RR et al. "Human head and neck kinematics after low velocity rear-end impacts-understanding 'Whiplash.'" 1995, SAE Paper 952724.

275. GOTTEN N. "Survey of 100 cases of whiplash injury after settlement of litigation." JAMA 1956; 162;865-867.

276. SCHUTT CH and DOHAN FC. 'Neck injury to women in auto accidents. A metropolitan plague." JAMA 1968;206:2689-2692.

277. NORRIS SH and WATT I. "The prognosis of neck injuries resulting from rear-end collisions." J Bone Joint Surg 1983; 65-B:608-611.

278. DEANS GT, MCGALLIARD JN, RUTHERFORD WH. "Incidence and duration of neck pain among patients injured in car accidents. Br Med J 1986;292:94-95.

279. LIVINGSTON M. "Whiplash injury and peer copying." J Roy Soc Med 1993;86:535-536.

280. LIVINGSTON M. "Whiplash injury:misconceptions and remedies." Aust Fam Phys 1992;21:1642-1647.

281. LIVINGSTON M. "Whiplash injury:some continuing problems." Humane Medicine 1993; 9:274-281.

282. FERRARI R. "The Whiplash Encyclopedia:The Facts and Myths of Whiplash. Maryland, Aspen Publishers Inc. 1999, 7, 253, 254.

283. MALLESON A. Whiplash and Other Useful Illnesses. Montreal, McGill-Queens University Press 2002, 26,28,485.

284. HOHL M. "Soft tissue injuries of the neck in automobile accidents; factors influencing prognosis. J Bone and Jt Surgery 1974; 56A:1675-1682.

285. PORTER KM. Editorial. "Neck sprains after car accidents;a common cause of long term disability." Brit Med J 1989;298:973-4.

286. CRAIG GL. "Sorting out the points of whiplash investigation." Can J Diagnosis 1992;9:95-107.

287. TEASELL R, MCCAIN GA, MERSKEY H and FINESTONE H. "Cervical sprain or whiplash: an often-rejected injury. Humane Med 1991; 7:183-7.

288. BLOCH R. "Methodology in clinical back pain trials." Spine 1987; 12:430-2.

289. MELVILLE PH. "Research in car crashing." [Letter] Can Med Assoc J 1963;89:275.

290. BERRY H. "Chronic whiplash syndrome as a functional disorder." Arch Neurol 2000 57:592-594.

291. TAYLOR JR and TWOMEY LT. "Acute injuries to cervical joints. An autopsy study of neck sprain." Spine 1993; 18:1115-1122.

292. BOGDUK N and TEASELL R. "Whiplash. The evidence for an organic etiology." Arch Neurol 2000;57: 590-591.

293. TEASELL RW and MERSKEY H. 'Whiplash injuries: A review." Verdict. 2001. Issue 89.52-65.

294. MILLS H and HORNE G. "Whiplash –man made disease." NZ Med J 1986; 99:373-374.

295. HORNE G. (C) "Neck sprains after car accidents." Br Med J 1989; 299:53.

296. AWERBACH MS. "Whiplash in Australia:illness or injury?" Med J Aust 1992;157:193-196.

297. BALLA JI. "The late whiplash syndrome: A study of an illness in Australia and Singapore." Culture Med Psychiatry 1982; 6: 191-210.

298. LIVINGSTON M. "Neck and back sprains from MVA's: a retrospective study." BC Med J 1991;33:654-656.

299. FERRARI R, RUSSELL AS. "The Whiplash Syndrome.

Commonsense revisited." [Editorial.] J Rheumatology 1997;24:623-625.

300. SULLIVAN M. "Whiplash: Can the cost to society be diminished?" In GUNZBERG R,SZPALSKI M. Whiplash Injuries. Current Concepts in Prevention, Diagnosis, and Treatment of Cervical Whiplash Syndrome. Philadelphia, Lippincott-Raven, 1998, p.331-333.

301. SPITZER WO et al. Quebec Task Force on Whiplash-Associated Disorders. Spine 1995; 20:Supp S 73.

302. SCHRADER H, OBELIENIENE D, BOVIM G, SURKIENE D, et al. "Natural evolution of the late whiplash syndrome outside the medical context." Lancet 1996; 347:1207-1211.

303. CASSIDY JD, CAROLL LJ, COTE P, LEMSTRA M, et al. "Effect of eliminating compensation for pain and suffering on the outcome of insurance claims for whiplash injury." N Engl J Med 2000; 342:1179-1186.

304. FREEMAN MD, CROFT AC, ROSSIGNOL AM, WEAVER DS, et al. "A review and methodologic critique of the literature refuting whiplash syndrome." Spine 1999;24:86-96.

305. OBELIEIENE D, SCHRADER H, BOVIM G et al. "Pain after whiplash-a prospective controlled inception cohort study." J Neurol Neurosurg Psychiatry 1999; 66:279-283.

306. PARTHENI M et al. "Whiplash injury." J Rheumatol 1999; 26: 1206-1207.

307. FERRARI R "Whiplash is a social disorder – How so!" BC Med J 2002;44:307-311.

308. TAYLOR JR. "The Pathology of Whiplash: Neck sprain." BC Med J 2002; 44:252-246.

309. RUSSELL AS. Foreword in Livingston M. Common Whiplash Injury: A Modern Epidemic. Springfield, Ill. Charles C. Thomas, 1999, v-vi.

310. GALASKO CSB. "Incidence of whiplash-associated disorder." BC Med J 2002; 44:237-240.

311. LIVINGSTON M. Common Whiplash Injury: A Modern Epidemic. Springfield, Ill. Charles C. Thomas, 1999, 158-159.

312. ALLEN M. "Whiplash claims and costs in British Columbia." BC Med J 2002; 44: 241-242.

313. HIPPOCRATES. "Epidemics I." In Hippocrates, Vol. 1. (Trans, by Jones WHS.) London: William Heineman, 1923. p.165.

314. HADLER N. Occupational Musculoskeletal Disorders. 3rd Ed. Philadelphia, Lippincott Williams & Wilkins. 2005. Preface to the First Edition, xi.

315. KWAN O, FRIEL J. "A review and methodologic critique of the literature supporting 'chronic whiplash injury.' Part 1 – research articles." Med Sci Mon 2003;9 (8): RA 203-215.

316. FERRARI R, SCHRADER H. "The late whiplash syndrome: a biopsychosocial approach." J Neurol Neurosurg Psychiatry 2001;70:722-726.

317. HUNTER KM. Doctors' Stories, The Narrative Structure of Medical Knowledge Princeton, Princeton University Press. 1991, p.103,105.

318. JUNG CG. "The Undiscovered self." In The Essential Jung. Coll. By Storra, Princeton, Princeton University Press. 1983. p. 349-403.

319. ENGEL GL. "The clinical application of the biopsychosocial model." Am J Psych 1980; 137:535-544.

320. ENGEL GL. "From biomedical to biopsychosocial: Being scientific in the human domain." Psychosomatics 1997; 38:521-528.

321. WISE TN. Editorial note in ENGEL GL. "From biomedical to biopsychosocial: Being scientific in the human domain." Psychosomatics 1997;38:521.

322. BECKMAN HB, FRANKEL RM. "The effect of physician

behaviour on the collection of data." Am Intern Med 1984; 101:692-696.

323. BRODY H. Stories of Sickness. New Haven and London. Yale University Press, 1987. p 188-189.

324. BAYLISS R. "Pain Narratives," in Narrative-Based Medicine. (Eds.) Trish Greenhalgh and Brian Hurwitz. Ibid. P. 75-82.

325. HUNTER KM. Doctors' Stories. Ibid. p. 169.

326. SHORTER E. From Paralysis to Fatigue. Ibid. p. 11.

327. SHAKESPEARE W. The First Part of the History of Henry iv. Cambridge, Cambridge University Press, 1968. Act 2, Scene 3, p. 31.

328. CHAN AW, HROBJARTSSON A, HAAHR MT, GOTZSCHE PC. et al. "Empirical evidence for selective reporting of outcomes in randomized trials: comparison of protocols to published articles." JAMA 2004; 291:2457-2465.

329. HADLER N. "Fibromyalgia: La maladie est morte: Vive le maladie!" [Editorial.] J Rheumatol 1997; 24:1250-1251.

330. BALINT M. Ibid. p. 108.

331. HADLER N. Ed. Clinical Concepts in Regional Musculoskeletal Illness. Orlando. Florida. Grune and Stratton, inc. 1988, p. 6.

332. WHITE KL, WILLIAMS TF, GREENBERG BG. "The ecology of medical care." NEJM 1961; 265:885-892.

333. FALK WA. The Curious Family Doctor. Research by family doctors in Canada in the early days. Victoria, BC Trafford Publishing. 2001.

334. HUTT P with HEATH I and NEIGHBOUR R. Confronting an Ill Society. David Widgery, General practice, idealism and the chase for change. Oxford, Radcliffe Publishing, 2005.

335. ROURKE JT. "An honour and a privilege." Can Fam Phys 2004;50:983.

ACKNOWLEDGEMENTS

It is difficult to acknowledge every individual or organization who has helped the publication of this work. I am grateful to be able to use some of my material previously published in the Australian family Physician, B.C. Medical Journal, Back Aid, George Stickley, Philadelphia, Canadian Family Physician, Canadian Medical Association Journal, Clinical Orthopedics, Common Whiplash Injury: A Modern Epidemic, Charles C Thomas, Pa; Family Medicine: an Inside Look, Orc Enterprises, Richmond, BC; Humane Medicine, J Family Practice, J Rheumatology, J Roy Soc Med, Lancet, Legal Medical Quarterly, Manual Medicine, Medical Journal of Australia, Orthopedic Research, The Practitioner, West J Med. I am also grateful to be able to use material from Henri Chatenay, The Country Doctors, Red Deer Albera, Mattrix Press; from Dr.John Coope, Dr Chekhov: A Study in Literature and Medicine, Isle of Wight, Cross Publishing, and H Troyat, Chekhov, New York, Random House; Helm M H and Karlinsky S, Letters of Anton Chekhov, New York, Harper & Row; Williams WC, The Autobiography of William Carlos Williams, New York, New Directions Publishing Corp; Williams WC, The Doctor Stories. New York, New Directions Publishing Corp; Mair, A, Sir James Mackenzie MD 1853-1925. General Practitioner. Edinburgh, Churchill Livingstone, Gunn C C, The Gunn Approach to the Treatment of Chronic Pain. New York, Churchill Livingston; Hunter K M, Doctors' Stories. The Narrative Structure of Medical Knowledge, Princeton, Princeton University Press; Balint M, The Doctor. His Patient and the Illness. Edinburgh, Churchill Livingstone.

I thank Peter Broomhall, Ian McWhinney, Bill Rivers, Alex Campbell, Alan Thackray, Chris Morrant, Jim Wilson, Galt Wilson,

Molly and Bill Falk, Donald Calne and Dr. Gavin Stuart, Dean of Medicine, University of British Columbia for their advice and help. Any Errors are mine. I thank my office nurses Brenda Martens and Fran Collard who for many years put patients at ease; also Fran for her suggestions, for patient typing and retyping of the manuscript, and my wife Diana for her patience and our sons John and Peter for their suggestions, and Peter for rescuing the manuscript. I thank Dr. Anthony Russell, University of Alberta, for kindly consenting to compose the foreword and the wonderful staff of the British Colmbia Medical Library for their continuing assistance.

Finally, I wish to thank Valerie Johnson and Julia Caranci, publishing consultants at Trafford Publishing for their advice, support and enthusiasm. Also Amber Huff, Alyx Gilgunn and staff at Trafford Publishing for speeding the work through to fruition.

AUTHOR INDEX

The number refers to the number in the text, not the page number.

SUBJECT INDEX

Abdominal surgery avoided, 10
Acupuncture, 190
Air Council, 199
Alternative medicine, 258
America, 138
American Grain, in the, 132
Amoebic dysentery, 228
Anecdotal cases, 32,33
Angina Pectoris, 174
Ann, dairymaid, 56
Anxiety, 31,38,84
Appendicitis, 14
Auto-injury claims, 32,34
Automobile demolition derby, 289
Autonomic dysfunction in
        back pain, 188

Balint, Michael, 335
Battle of Britain, the, 200
Bella Coola Valley, BC 183
Berry, Henry, 290
Bone-setter, 22
Bornholm disease, 147
Brasset, Edmund, 180
British Columbia,
        27,183, 198, 239, 311
British Columbia Medical
Journal, 307
British Columbia, University of,
        239
British Medical Journal, 22

Burnley, 75

Cambridge University, 198
Cancer, fear of, 31
Canso, Nova Scotia, 180
Case notes, records, 35,59,64,324
Cervical collar, overuse, 2
Cervical spine, 1
Chekhov, Anton,
        65,67,69,71,73,89,107
Childbirth, 32
    case of 'Doc' Williams, 131
    case of Dr. Mackenzie, 164
Chiropractic,
        22,23,24,25,26,202,205
Cholera, 108
Chorea, 60
Chronic whiplash syndrome,
        38,289,305,306

Clinical Orthopedics,23
Common whiplash injury,
(cervical sprain)
Biomechanics of,
        30,271,272,273,274
Book, 68

Compensation and, 294,296,300
Confusion in, 38,306,315
Copying patterns in,
        277,279,280,281

218

ISBN 141207169-0